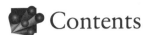 Contents

· GENERAL · PRACTICE

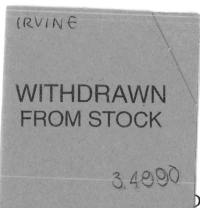

Making Sense of Audit

SECOND EDITION

EDITED BY
DONALD and SALLY IRVINE

FOREWORD BY
SIR KENNETH CALMAN

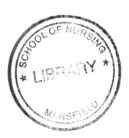

DICAL PRESS

© 1997 Donald and Sally Irvine

Radcliffe Medical Press Ltd
18 Marcham Road, Abingdon, Oxon OX14 1AA, UK

Reprinted 1997

First edition 1991

British Library Cataloguing in Publication Data

A catalogue record for this book is available from the British Library.

ISBN 1 85775 119 1

Library of Congress Cataloging-in-Publication Data is available.

Typeset by Acorn Bookwork, Salisbury, Wiltshire
Printed and bound by Biddles Ltd, Guildford and King's Lynn

Foreword

THERE is little doubt that quality of health care is at the heart of the health service agenda. No matter how difficult it is to define quality, we need ways of ensuring that it is monitored and continually improved. Quality is a relative concept in that there is always a reference to standards and, as standards are always rising, this implies that it can always be improved. Audit is one way in which the quality of care can be assessed. It is a tool which can be used with great advantage but, as with all tools, requires regular honing to keep it sharp and effective. Its objective is to contribute to improving the care of patients.

Audit is not new. It has been part of clinical practice for generations. What has changed has been its formalization within the health service and the national imperative to consider its practice in a more systematic way. It is perhaps this which has encouraged a certain mystique around audit with high priests and priestesses, gurus and experts. This has tended to emphasize the specialist nature of audit rather than its general applicability. This book takes as its starting point that all doctors can, and should, be involved.

Doctors, and other professionals, learn by telling stories to each other. These tales, generally known as case presentations, are presented to colleagues for advice, comment and questioning. In long winter evenings saga are told of difficult problems overcome by wisdom, experience and great technical skill. Occasionally such stories are collected together and told to a wider audience through journals and books. Audit, as a process, allows these individual stories to be collected in a systematic way and compared and connected to the wider literature, one of the reference sources for standards. Audit allows the clinical practice of an individual, or a group, to be related to standards and quality indicators defined by the individual or group itself, or by reference to others. In addition to comparing one practice with another, practice may be changed as a result of the process. It is this part of audit, sometimes called 'closing the loop', which provides the audit process with its power to modify and improve standards.

The case studies in this book add a very practical dimension about how to put audit into practice. While each individual example may not be relevant to every reader, they provide an insight into the way of thinking about audit and its consequences. They represent a splendid collection of stories. There is no substitute, however, for getting started and doing it.

Finally, this book is called *Making Sense of Audit*. It is about making it understandable, and putting it in context. But the use of the word 'sense' is also important. All of our senses have afferent and efferent loops. There is a central organ for the synthesis of information with action which follows if it is appropriate. What a good model for clinical audit. But there is another way in which the term may be used, and that is as in 'commonsense'. This remains a very important part of the practice of audit, and this book shows how this commonsense can be applied to improving the care of patients.

KENNETH CALMAN
APRIL 1997

List of contributors

JAMES COX, MD, FRCGP, MICGP, *General Practitioner, Caldbeck, Cumbria; formerly Associate Adviser in General Practice, University of Newcastle upon Tyne*

PAUL CREIGHTON, FRCGP, *General Practitioner, Coquet Medical Group, Broomhill, Northumberland; Associate Adviser in General Practice, University of Newcastle upon Tyne*

LYNN GRAHAM, LLB, ACA, *Practice Manager, Guidepost Medical Group, Northumberland*

ALLEN HUTCHINSON, FRCGP, *Professor in Public Health Medicine, University of Hull; formerly General Practitioner, Lintonville Medical Group, Ashington, Northumberland*

SIR DONALD IRVINE, CBE, MD, FRCGP, President, General Medical Council; formerly General Practitioner, Lintonville Medical Group, Ashington, Northumberland and Regional Adviser in General Practice, University of Newcastle upon Tyne

SALLY IRVINE, MA (Cantab), FRCGP (Hon), FAMGP Professional Practice Consultant, formerly General Administrator, Royal College of General Practitioners, London; Vice-President, Association of Health Centre and Practice Administrators

COLIN LEON, MBE, FRCGP, *formerly General Practitioner, Gateshead, Tyne and Wear; formerly Associate Adviser in General Practice, University of Newcastle upon Tyne*

GEORGE TAYLOR, FRCGP, MICGP, DRCOG, *General Practitioner, Guidepost Medical Group, Northumberland; Associate Adviser in General Practice, University of Newcastle upon Tyne*

ROGER THORNHAM, FRCGP, *General Practitioner, Norton Medical Centre, Stockton-on-Tees; Associate Adviser in General Practice, University of Newcastle upon Tyne*

Acknowledgements

WE are extremely grateful to the practices of all the contributors for allowing their colleagues to draw freely on their experiences of audit, and for allowing us to use new material where relevant.

The staff of the Division for General Practice within the Postgraduate Institute for Medicine and Dentistry in the University of Newcastle upon Tyne, together with our personal assistants, Lesley Loach and Anne Whersley, have been helpful and supportive throughout, and we thank them.

DONALD AND SALLY IRVINE
APRIL 1997

Section I

1 Introduction

AUDIT is the process used by health professionals to assess, evaluate and improve the care of patients in a systematic way in order to enhance their health and quality of life.

The first part of this book (Section I) is a description of audit. There is an account of its basic benefits and uses, and of the methods available to carry it out. The essential data requirements of different types of audit are discussed, as is the analysis of results, and how to bring about change in a practice where the results of audit suggest it is appropriate to do so.

The reader could stop there. However, Section II continues with a collection of case histories from the contributors' general practices. Each case history summarizes a working audit of a particular practice which was carried out to help overcome practical problems and to secure improvements. The strength of the case histories lies in their simplicity. They show what worthwhile things can be done with a little thought and imagination, the expenditure of a modest amount of effort and money, and with the use of knowledge and skills which are available in every practice. Those who have previously felt daunted by the mystique of audit – that it is something rarefied and special – may take encouragement from them!

The case histories, and the examples cited in the opening chapters, show how general practices, wanting to provide a good quality of service to their patients, see audit as indispensable to the delivery of patient care, as for example, the medical records system. Audit can help simplify the organization of work and so take some of the stress out of life. It can show whether or not a practice is achieving what it set out to do. It has the potential to be one of the most important factors in improving the health of the practice community, and can lead to changes which result in patients being more content with the service they receive. Audit can also show conscientious doctors, nurses, receptionists and other staff where their professional knowledge and skills could be strengthened.

Audit in context

Ten years ago, clinical audit in general practice was still the prerogative of enthusiasts who enjoyed looking at their work in a structured and objective way. Some went a step further, using practice data to compare themselves with other practices, to see where they stood in the wider world. For these doctors and their practices the benefits of audit were self-evident, and the value of audit was demonstrated to them time and again through their experience with it.

Seven years ago the Government institutionalized clinical audit as part of the health reforms, and since then has spent considerable sums of money trying to establish it in both general and hospital specialty practice. In general practice the Medical Audit Advisory Groups (MAAG) were set up to assist with implementation. The general feeling, which the authors share, is that the MAAG and equivalent local audit groups have done a very good job. They seem to have been more successful than their hospital counterparts, perhaps because they have tried to be 'user friendly', helping practices to understand audit and to get started in ways that they can handle. They are an excellent source of practical advice.

Despite this investment, however, and the best efforts of the MAAG, a general feeling persists that audit has somehow failed fully to capture the hearts and minds of many doctors, and has hardly touched the non-medical health professions in primary care. There is clearly a gap between the expectations of policy makers on the one hand and the attitudes of some practitioners on the other. There are several reasons for this mismatch, some professional and some managerial. For example, the rhetoric of the medical profession has tended to present clinical audit primarily as an educational experience separate from everyday practice. National Health Service (NHS) management has tended to reinforce this rather detached approach by linking audit in doctors' minds with wider policies on cost containment, efficiency savings and the like – not the most popular of motivators for health professionals.

Yet reality, as is shown in this book, is different again. Whatever one's feelings, audit is here to stay. The health professions and NHS management are both determined to establish evidence-based practice, to ensure as far as possible that health care is clinically effective – that is, it is safe, based on the best research available, and beneficial – and that it gives value for money. Clinical audit, because it relates current practice to given standards, has therefore become one of the essentials for health professionals in a society which expects patient-oriented care, explicit standards, demonstrable effectiveness, regular improvement and visible accountability from its health providers. Clinical audit is now mainstream general practice. It is no longer an optional extra.

Audit and practice management

Modern general practices are about teamwork. They are beginning to develop the habit of collective responsibility. Therefore, they are becoming used to working with practice development plans and seeing these as an important device to help them determine their future direction. It is from this capacity to plan, and a willingness to look ahead, that they derive their objectives for care, identify the clinical and operational criteria and standards that indicate good care, and decide on the main activities necessary to achieve them. They monitor what is done to make things happen as planned. This process of defining clinical and operational objectives and standards, and of monitoring and assessing progress towards them, is known as the management cycle.

The methods and techniques used to carry out simple practice audits follow exactly the same principles as are used in the management cycle in general practice. Indeed, they become part and parcel of the same thing. Both require the collection and analysis of practice data, and the comparison of the results against what are understood to be or have been explicitly stated as the practice's objectives for care.

Audit may indicate the need for change. Management is the process within a practice whereby change is achieved. Audit can be a powerful and effective aid for bringing about change in an acceptable and workable manner, because it provides reliable, up-to-date facts about a practice and its performance, the starting point for effective decision making. The neutrality and objectivity of performance data may be especially valuable where the reasons for making changes may not be obvious to or accepted by all members of the practice team, especially where it is going to involve demanding or uncomfortable adjustments by some individuals.

A key to quality

Audit and management are complementary, interlocking functions. They are two of the basic building blocks that the modern practice team must use if it wants to ensure the quality of its care. Using audit helps a practice team to understand and acknowledge the extent to which one member is dependent on the quality of the work of others, and the degree of accountability that all members of the team have to the people who are registered with their practice. Personal self-sufficiency, self-reliance and self-discipline are all attributes associated with quality care and quality management.

The case studies reveal how these attributes appeal to health professionals who are keen to exercise considerable freedom of responsibility in the care of patients, without excessive direction from outside. Experience has shown that, in general terms, practice teams that have a positive approach to quality are more likely to be happy and confident in what they do, and are more likely to secure the funding they seek for practice developments they think are important.

This book aims to present audit in as straightforward, logical and understandable a way as possible. It is written with every member of the practice team in mind, although the partners, as proprietors, have a pivotal role in giving leadership. The companion book, *The Practice of Quality*,[1] sets audit in the wider context of quality-minded teamworking and quality improvement in general practice. It will be helpful reading for general practitioners, registrars, nurses and practice managers who want to know how they can best ensure that their practices succeed in the new environment of a primary care-led NHS.

2 The benefits of audit: why do it?

ATTITUDES to audit are undoubtedly coloured by the way people think it will be used. For example, when audit is presented as an aid to education it is generally seen by the medical profession in a positive light – i.e. a 'good thing'. On the other hand, when audit is perceived as an instrument of health service management, perhaps to check on work done or to cut costs, it is more likely to be seen as a threat because the results may lead to imposed change.

Actually, audit is relatively easy to understand and carry out. The main difficulties are in generating the interest and commitment to do it in the first place and, subsequently, in handling change where the need is demonstrated. Motivation is clearly tied up with purpose and the use to which audit will be put. This chapter is at the heart of the 'why bother?' argument. Bringing about change, which involves the often delicate process of altering behaviour in oneself and others, is described in more detail in Chapter 10.

To be clear about purpose, audit must be seen in its wider context. The NHS has two main functions: to provide care to individual patients and to secure improvements in the health of the community. These functions are being carried out at a time when modern medicine can do more than ever for people – at a cost – and when the public's expectations of service have never been higher. Hence the drive to refocus the NHS on patients rather than the providers of health care,[1] and on making care as clinically effective and practically efficient as possible.[2,3]

The practice of evidence-based, clinically effective health care is fast becoming one of the 'givens' of general practice today.[4,5] Audit is one of the essential tools that enables practices to know whether they are giving effective care. This is why its status is no longer negotiable. The real question, therefore, is how best to help members of practice teams to get to grips with this reality in ways that they see will make life better for them, as well as which meet their patients' and society's expectations. Enlightened self-interest is one of life's most powerful motivators.

Taking control

Some practices, with enlightened self-interest very much in mind, have decided that they, rather than health authority managers, must steer, influence and control their everyday work with patients. Anecdotal evidence suggests that practices which feel they are in charge of their own destinies are happy and successful. Their success depends very substantially on the extent to which they are able to use performance data, gained through audit, to show what they are doing and how well. Audit data empower them by providing detailed knowledge about their patients and the performance of their teams, which health authority managers do not have. For them, audit has become one of the drivers of the practice, and one of the safeguards of their independence.

On the other hand, there are general practitioners who feel that in today's NHS they have lost control over their professional lives and their practices. Much of their demoralization, lack of confidence and the sense of being overwhelmed by rising demand can be attributed to this loss of control. These practices, if they use audit at all, see it as an imposition from outside, another chore to be added to a list of activities that they do not see as relevant to mainline care. Lacking both a sense of direction and the means to steer their own course, they have no option but to be swept along with the tide.

So, knowledge is power and audit is the source of exclusive knowledge about the work of an individual practice. Successful practices understand this, which is why audit is so important to them. The practical benefits of audit to such practices are listed in Box 2.1. They are what the contributors have identified to be the most important benefits in improving care for their patients and the quality of their professional lives. The list is by no means exhaustive, nor is it set in any particular order. Nor are the divisions between the benefits discrete. Indeed, members of a practice will want to make up their own lists of desired benefits. Such discussion will in itself help practice teams to be sure of their reasons for performing audit.

Box 2.1: Audit: the practical benefits

A practice can use audit to:

- reduce frustration, hassle and stress
- help get a grip on workload
- demonstrate good care
- improve effectiveness
- improve efficiency
- reduce clinical and organizational error
- improve patient satisfaction
- promote education
- bid for resources
- manage risk

Reducing frustration

The most immediate and obvious benefit of audit is its value in helping to alleviate or remove those burdens of everyday practice that can be so frustrating. This can be a very persuasive motivator when some partners are sceptical about the value of audit. Every practice has problems that everyone complains about, but which no one seems able to solve. By defining, quantifying and analysing a problem through audit, solutions may emerge which can then be tried, tested, and then reassessed for their effectiveness in subsequent audits. Two simple yet familiar situations are presented in Examples 2.1 and 2.2.

Example 2.1

A practice had a problem with missing case notes. The receptionists decided to keep a record of the places where these notes were eventually found. As a result of a month's simple audit changes were made to the movement of patient notes, using tracer cards more effectively, a computerized tracker system – and a daily clearing of the car boots of the partners until they learnt not to leave them there!

Example 2.2

A medical group was very frustrated by an apparent increase in the number of patients who were failing to attend for surgery appointments. This was resulting in longer surgeries as more extras were being slotted in, and was causing unacceptable delays in patients getting appointments within the practice's standard of 48 hours for routine consultations.

The partners decided to audit the 'did not attends' (DNAs) over a one-month period. Each patient who missed an appointment without cancelling was followed up by telephone, or a personal interview when they next attended surgery, using a structured questionnaire. The data showed:

- who the DNAs were
- the patterns of non-attendance
- reasons for non-attendance
- reasons for not cancelling the appointment.

The data were used as the basis for a practice strategy for coping with the problem. A further audit showed where there had been improvement.

Case study 10 gives a more comprehensive example of a practice which used the appointment of a new manager to find out what was causing frustration and irritation within a practice team.

Getting a grip on workload

Almost every general practice has its own experience of workload problems. These are invariably stressful and not always easy to solve, because the solutions may involve change which can affect the way of life or the way of working of individuals, and probably incur considerable expense.

In these situations much time and energy may be spent on discussing the need for change with little idea of how to bring it about. The difficulty may be compounded if only one or two partners seek change. Accurate written descriptions of the current position, and data derived from a practice audit, can show a way forward. Examples 2.3 and 2.4 provide familiar illustrations.

Example 2.3

The new young partner in a busy inner-city practice felt overwhelmed by the workload he had inherited from the retiring senior partner. After three months he complained to his three partners, who were themselves very pressed and felt unable to take any load from him. The oldest partner reassured the young man that he would speed up as he got more experienced, and the receptionists tried to keep the extras away from him.

At the end of nine months he was complaining daily about the workload and at the inequity of his partnership share. The other partners continued to ignore the problem, putting it down to the fact that he seemed to be a slow, even neurotic consulter. They felt that their new partner added to their own workloads, a feeling reinforced when the new partner made it clear that he would not feel able to take on any management responsibility in the practice for the foreseeable future.

Relationships and morale sank to an all-time low, until the practice manager suggested they should carry out an audit of workload, in terms of patient list profiles, consultation rates, return consultation figures and so on. After some initial reservations the partners agreed to do this. The results showed that the new partner had indeed a heavy workload, as the inherited list had a significantly higher number of elderly, chronically sick patients. The style and pattern of the retired partner had led to highly dependent behaviours in his patients, which the new partner was not experienced enough to correct. This aggravated his inherently slower consultation rate.

On the basis of these facts the partners were able to look at the workload problem with a fresh and more sympathetic eye. Prejudice and preconceived assumptions had given a distorted view of the true situation. They decided that a part-time assistant was needed to give them all some relief.

Example 2.4

The partners of a busy practice in a depressed inner-city area felt demoralized by their inability to handle the working day efficiently. Time for patients was too often foreshortened, patients complained too often about long waiting times for routine appointments, and receptionists tended to get caught between pressed doctors and irritated patients. At various times the problem was said to be:

- a higher than average patient demand
- the impact of outside appointments on doctor availability in the practice
- an inflexible way of organizing surgeries
- too little time for the average consultation (six minutes)
- a higher than average list size
- an unspoken perception that some partners worked harder than others
- an uncritical approach to delegation

All of these factors may have been contributory causes. Various *ad hoc*, stop-gap measures were tried without success. Eventually, in exasperation, the decision was made to collect prospective data on consultation patterns and patient demand for appointments from both the doctors and practice nurses, relating these to a predetermined 'ideal' standard time for consultations (ten minutes) and doctor availability. In the event the partnership was able to see, for the first time, exactly what was happening and how wide the gap actually was between the current position and the ideal that the partners were aiming for.

A quite new organization of medical and nursing work resulted in more time for patients which, the partners would now freely concede, seemed unattainable previously. Subsequent audits were used with enthusiasm to fine-tune the new arrangements, gaining even more improvements.

Example 2.4 illustrates the important point that fitful, knee-jerk attempts at systematic relief seldom work – on the contrary, they can reinforce a feeling of hopelessness that the problem really is insuperable. It shows equally that audit data can help to build up an accurate picture of reality, from which a diagnosis can be made and possible solutions identified. Case studies 8 and 9 are further examples.

Demonstrating good care

Demonstrating good care is one of the traditional uses of audit. However, there is some argument about whether this is the best use of a practice's time and resources.

Those who favour demonstrating good care argue that it is insufficient for a practice team to feel that it does its job well: the quality of service should be there for all to see. The demonstration of good care can boost a practice team's morale, enabling it to feel valued and valuable. Case study 7 shows how such an audit can be done simply, in this instance by using a 'tracer' condition (*see* Chapter 7).

Those who are against the demonstration of good care argue that it deflects energy from problems where there is considerable scope for improvement. However, if auditors always focus upon things that appear to be wrong, it can have a depressing effect. The practice team is probably best served by attempting to achieve a judicious balance in its selection of subjects.

Being effective

As clinically effective practice is the objective, there is a new sense of urgency to integrate the results of proven research more quickly into individual patient care. In essence, this means using methods of investigation and treatment which have demonstrable value in terms of efficacy, and stopping doing things which have no such value.

Clinical effectiveness relates directly to clinical outcome. It demonstrates the extent to which a practice's objectives for improving patients' health care are met. Case studies 1, 5 and 12 show this.

Example 2.5 also shows the impact of external stimuli to resolve a problem already identified, and the futility of performing audits when a practice does not act on the results, even when it is clear about the direction in which it wants to go.

Example 2.5

A busy urban practice, which had many deprived children registered with it, accepted the need for effective immunization in childhood. The immunization rate was seen by the partners as an appropriate measure of success, as its high degree of acquired immunity would eliminate the infections against which protection was being given.

Despite this acceptance, periodic audits over several years showed less than optimum immunization rates. Lack of improvement was largely attributed to the difficulty of gaining access to some of the deprived children. However, it became obvious that this was being used as an excuse: the practice's tracking systems were found to be inadequate and the working practices inflexible. Furthermore, no single person had been assigned responsibility for implementing an immunization programme, and therefore no one was accountable.

The new contracting arrangements in general practice provided an outside stimulus to assign responsibility for the programme, to sort out the system and to find new ways of ensuring that children who had defaulted previously were immunized. Further audits showed a progressive improvement, such that the practice was able to meet its contract target rates comfortably.

Periodic audits have now been abandoned in favour of continuous performance monitoring, so that the practice knows exactly where it stands on a day-to-day basis. The current immunization rate for children under two years of age is 94%.

Improving efficiency

Effective care should be linked with efficient care to secure the best possible result with the most economical use of people, time and money. In the new climate of contracting and commissioning, or whatever variants of these may follow in the next few years, practices that can demonstrate effective and efficient care will be much better placed to bid for the resources they need to do the job well. By contrast, practices that cannot articulate their requirements are almost bound to be less successful. In making the most efficient use of resources, audits have an important function in practice management and can yield worthwhile improvements (*see* Examples 2.6, 2.7 and 2.8). In Case study 1, audit was used to improve the efficiency of an 'over-75' screening programme, and in Case study 14 it was employed to assess the efficiency of a rubella immunization programme.

Example 2.6

In an urban practice, an audit of routine data on patterns of doctor-initiated surgery attendances revealed a significant variation among partners in the rates of 'return' consultations. This variation could not be accounted for by differences in the demographic characteristics of patients attending or the nature of the illnesses. A further audit pinpointed the main cause, which was the difference in the basis on which each doctor decided whether and when patients should return.

Using this information, the partners reviewed their decision-making process and formulated guidelines to ensure more consistency in future. Subsequent monitoring (or audit) showed that one partner had increased the return rate, two had not altered their rate and three had reduced it. The new basis for bringing patients back was thought to be more appropriate – at least it could be better justified – and the overall return rate was reduced, reflecting an improvement in efficiency.

Example 2.7

A practice manager, noting the time it took for some partners to send off 'short reports', initiated a simple, prospective audit designed to show the time lapse between receipt of the request and despatch of the report, partner by partner.

The partners were surprised at how long the delays were, and thereby became aware of the potential loss of income to the practice. An explicit protocol to ensure prompt return was introduced, and the practice manager was asked to continue periodic audits, to make sure there was no backsliding.

Example 2.8

A practice was concerned at the number of times patients returned to the surgery for X-ray reports which were not actually available. A short, prospective audit was carried out to find out why.

The results, and related enquiries, showed that the causes of the delay were the length of time it took for the reports to be typed in the hospital typing pool, and an inefficient filing system in the practice office. As a consequence, the practice defined explicit operational standards for its own office, but it found it difficult to influence the hospital. Subsequent check audits showed improvement in the practice office, but none at the hospital.

Later, the practice became a fundholder and used its purchasing power to bring about an improved hospital response.

Reducing error

Conscientious health professionals are interested in trying to reduce or eliminate the chances of clinical and organizational error. Mishaps can occur either as a result of a single failure, such as a missed diagnosis or the wrong choice of treatment, or repeatedly, because of a flaw in a practice system or through lack of competence or persistently deficient performance. Periodic audits can help to show where these errors occur.

Both clinical and organizational errors have a direct impact on patient management. Boxes 2.2 and 2.3 give some examples of sources of error of each. In Case study 11 a confidential enquiry method of audit was used to reduce both types of error.

Box 2.2: Sources of clinical error

- Failure to check on the extent to which therapeutic serum levels are actually achieved and maintained, for example in the drug treatment of thyroid deficiency and epilepsy.
- Clinical management situations, such as determining whether action is always taken on abnormal HbA levels in diabetic patients, or significant elevation of the blood pressure in hypertensive patients.
- Inappropriate delays in the diagnosis of life-threatening or potentially disabling diseases.

Box 2.3: Common sources of organizational error

- Faulty recall systems, leading to patients being missed.
- Absence of clear routines for handling reports: for example, positive cervical smear reports may be filed before action is taken, so that follow-up is delayed and patients damaged.
- Patients on long-term drug therapy using repeat prescriptions can be lost to follow-up if there is no effective system for triggering review.
- Inadequate access arrangements, leading to particularly dangerous delays.

There may be other benefits in reducing error. For instance, the efforts involved may bring a practice team closer together by promoting a better understanding between members. When every member of the team takes responsibility for meeting the challenge to minimize error a collective responsibility for quality and standards is the result.

Improving patient satisfaction

The use of surveys of patient expectations and satisfaction is becoming more common. They can reveal patterns of patient preference from which standards can be formulated, as Case study 3 and Example 2.9 demonstrate.

Example 2.9

A practice sought the advice of patients about the process of obtaining repeat prescriptions. Open-ended questions were asked, and resulted in some unexpected answers. For instance, patients showed that they would prefer not to come to the surgery, but would rather have their prescriptions sent to them in a stamped addressed envelope, which they were prepared to supply.

Patients expect doctors to provide a service which they feel will improve their health, and to do it in ways they think they would prefer. They see audits which engage their interest as evidence of a practice that cares.

Promoting education

Audit can yield educational benefits for a practice team. Some of these are set out in Box 2.4. As there is growing emphasis on questions of competence and performance, targeting education to the real service needs of individual practitioners is becoming ever more important.

Box 2.4: The educational benefits of audit

- Feedback to individual practitioners on personal performance, leading to ready identification of gaps in knowledge and skill.
- Stimulation for a group of partners or primary care teams to review current practice, standards and criteria. Case studies 1, 4, 8, 10 and 13 give examples of this, where additional learning potential and needs within the practice team have been revealed.
- Generating clinical guidelines through peer-group activity, or the assessment of the results and implication of audits carried out on each other.

Bidding for resources

The point about the value of efficiency was made earlier. Today the competition for available resources is keener than ever, which means that practices must be able to demonstrate the range, quality and cost of their services in order to attract money for new services, or resources to improve existing ones. Similarly, effective quality assurance, incorporating audit, will be important in securing funds for the introduction of new ideas and technology to help develop the practice.

Risk management

Clinical audit is now deemed by the medical profession to be part of good practice, a specific professional responsibility.[6] Nurses and other health professionals are sure to see it similarly in due course. In future, general practitioners who find themselves the subject of GMC enquiries into their performance, and who cannot offer coherent explanations for any seriously deficient pattern of performance, may place their registration and therefore their livelihood at risk.

Clinical and organizational audit offer doctors protection. By knowing their business well, by being able to describe their results, clearly, thoroughly and systematically, doctors will be better able to protect themselves against legal, regulatory or managerial action by being able to take preventative action before harm is done to patients. Practices without such early warning systems will be at a disadvantage, because they are less likely to know about trouble ahead until it is too late.

Conclusion

Clinical audit will always be an intellectually stimulating and enjoyable part of practice for the enthusiast, but these will always be in a minority. Far more important is the necessity of recognizing reality, i.e. that clinical and operational audit is now very much part and parcel of modern general practice. The key thing is to accept this fact, then use audit energetically in ways which will confer as much benefit as possible on health professionals and patients alike.

3   What is audit?

Definitions

AUDIT, as defined in Chapter 1, is the 'process used by health professionals to assess, evaluate and improve the care of patients in a systematic way, to enhance their health and quality of life'. It consists of four basic steps, which are summarized in Box 3.1 and shown in Fig. 3.1.

Box 3.1: Steps in audit

1 Identifying or defining criteria and standards, in order to answer the question 'What are we trying to achieve for our patients?'
2 Collecting data on current performance, i.e. the care given and its effects on patients.
3 Assessing performance against criteria and standards to determine the extent to which criteria and standards have been met.
4 Identifying the need for change, either to the way care is provided or to the criteria and standards.

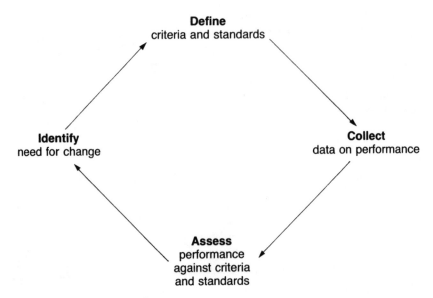

Figure 3.1   The audit cycle

This process of setting criteria and standards, monitoring perform-ance, and identifying and initiating appropriate change is known as the audit cycle; it should be repeated as necessary to ensure progressive improvement.

The characteristics of audit described above are found in most modern definitions (*see* Box 3.2).

Box 3.2: Some definitions of audit

1 The Quality Initiative of the Royal College of General Practitioners (RCGP, 1985)[1] asked doctors to:

- specify the services they provide
- define objectives for patient care
- assess their performance against these objectives
- where appropriate, change clinical practice.

2 The Department of Health (DoH) White Paper *Working for Patients* (1989)[2] defined medical audit as 'the systematic, critical analysis of the quality of medical care, including the procedures used for diagnosis and treatment, the use of resources, and the resulting outcome and quality of life for the patient'.

3 Shaw and Costain (1989)[3] described medical audit as 'a systematic approach to the peer review of medical care in order to identify opportunities for improvement and provide a mechanism for realising them'.

4 Hughes and Humphrey (1990)[4] summarized the essential features of audit in general practice as:

- defining standards, criteria, targets or protocols for good practice against which performance can be compared
- systematic gathering of objective evidence about performance
- comparing results against standards and/or among peers
- identifying deficiencies and taking action to remedy them
- monitoring the effects of action on quality.

The term 'audit' is frequently used as a synonym for 'quality assessment' or 'quality assurance'. Quality assessment is 'the comparison of care against predetermined standards'.[5] Quality assurance requires action to be taken on any deficiencies revealed by quality assessment.[6] Audit that requires change is therefore comparable with quality assurance and also contributes to it.

The value of questioning and justification

Audit stimulates doctors to ask questions about their work, to justify their actions to themselves and to their colleagues, and to modify their performance when necessary.

The examples of audit given in Chapter 2 and in the case studies suggest that 'auditors' should have a questioning frame of mind:

- What happened?
- Could we have done better?
- What does quality mean for this patient?

Self-questioning is a characteristic possessed by most professional people. It helps them to be as sure as possible that they have appropriate knowledge and skills, and that they perform as well as possible. It requires self-discipline, and is best carried out in the company of working colleagues so that each individual may be stimulated by interaction.

The practice team that makes time to question its direction, values and specific aspects of care will welcome audit. A questioning attitude will help to define a team's objectives and standards, bring about change, and explore new ground.

The principle of justification is equally central to the practice of medicine:

- Can I justify the treatment I ordered for this patient?
- I think I should have seen that baby last night; can I, then, justify having given advice over the telephone?

In ordinary life clinicians tend to follow accepted patterns of 'good practice', for example in establishing a diagnosis, or in organizing care. Significant departures from accepted patterns of practice have to be explained and subsequently justified; audit can provide data which might show what happened and why.

A framework for assessing care

Audit requires a framework in which the description, measurement, comparison and evaluation of the quality of health care can be made. Donabedian (1996)[7] proposed that the quality of health care be regarded as comprising three interrelated parts, called structure, process and outcome (Fig. 3.2).

Structure ⟶ Process ⟶ Outcome

Figure 3.2   A framework for assessing care

Structure

The term 'structure' describes the physical attributes of health care, such as the surgery building, practice equipment, the number and kind of people in the practice team, and the patient records. Common sense suggests that health care is likely to be more effective if it is carried out in comfortable surroundings with the right equipment, and by the most appropriate people.

Although the presence of desirable structural attributes does not of itself ensure that the individual doctor or nurse will give good care, better care is more likely. For example, the doctors in a practice may have an electro-cardiograph: its presence does not guarantee that they will use it appropriately, but if it was not present there would be no electrocardiograms to assist in diagnosis. The absence of appropriate structure, as in some practices situated in deprived areas, can diminish the chances of providing optimum care, even though competent doctors can give good care to some patients under adverse conditions. In other words, the structural features of a practice comprising the environment for care can promote quality or impede it.

The advantage of assessing the structural characteristics of care is that they are tangible and can therefore be counted, thereby making audit easy. The earliest audit studies of British general practice were mainly concerned with structure. Audits were used most effectively in the new training practices of the 1970s to describe and assess such features as premises, equipment, staff and teaching facilities at a time when these varied widely. As a result, explicit criteria and standards governing the physical environment of teaching practices were laid down, such that trainees could expect a consulting room of their own, a practice library with an appropriate collection of books, and a basic order to patient records. These and similar standards can be reaudited to ensure that the practices involved in teaching young doctors are continuing to provide an environment most likely to facilitate learning.

Thus, the presence of structural attributes increases the chance of good quality care, but does not ensure it. Structure, however, does not describe the performance of the health professional giving care; this is a fundamental weakness, and the reason why audits of structure are performed less often now.

Today, quality is assessed primarily on the basis of a doctor's performance, which embodies Donabedian's two other constituents of quality – process and outcome.

Process

The term 'process' describes the care given by a practitioner, i.e. what that practitioner does, the sum of actions and decisions that describe a person's professional practice. Doctors and nurses tend to identify the process of care with quality, because it describes what they do for their patients: it reflects their attitudes, knowledge and skill. Unlike structure, the process of care usually relates directly to the benefits patients derive as a result.

Studies of process – mainly of practice activity – may suggest better ways of doing things in the light of the most recent knowledge available. Audits of practice activities have investigated important aspects of care, such as prescribing habits, hospital referrals, laboratory and X-ray use, and patterns of clinical decision making. Most of the case studies in Section II are process audits.

Outcome

Donabedian defined 'outcome' as the changes in a patient's current and future health status that can be attributed to antecedent health care. Outcomes are therefore the definitive indicators of health; they describe the effectiveness of care: for example, did the patient survive a potentially fatal condition, or were the effects of a potentially disabling condition prevented or alleviated?

Measures of outcome are more difficult to achieve than those of process, especially in general practice, where so many conditions cannot be defined or diagnosed with precision. Some broad areas of outcome, decided upon by a consensus group of general practitioners, are shown in Box 3.3. These areas would have to be much more specific to become measurable entities.

Box 3.3: Measures of outcomes

- Prevention of disease or control of the disease process.
- Improvement or preservation of the patient's level of function in the family, at work, and in social activities.
- Relief of the patient's symptoms, distress and anxiety, and avoidance of iatrogenic symptoms.
- Prevention of premature death.
- Minimizing the cost of the illness to patient and family.
- Patient satisfaction with care provided.
- Relief or clarification of the patient's interpersonal problems.
- Preserving the patient's integrity from an ethical point of view.

Source: Buck, Fry and Irvine (1974)[8]

In selecting outcome measures the natural history of the disease has to be taken into account. For example, the care given to a patient with a minor virus infection would not be worth assessing because the condition is self-limiting – the outcome is predetermined and not related to any care given. Furthermore, the outcomes of chronic disease may not be apparent for many years, in which case it may be difficult to determine the contribution that care has made to outcome compared with the many other factors that could have had an effect.

Intermediate outcomes

Much time and energy has been spent in arguing the relative validity, reliability, feasibility and cost of process and outcome measures as expressions of the quality of health care. Good measures of outcome are difficult to identify because it is hard to distinguish between the effects of antecedent care and other factors that may have influenced the patient's condition; the length of time that may have elapsed between giving care and its effects on the patient can also distort the suitability of outcome measures. Process measures are more suitable because they are immediate and easier to quantify; however, there is not always a causal relationship between care given (process) and the effects on the patient (outcome). For example, the prescription of the appropriate antibiotic (process) may be expected to shorten the period of disability (outcome) caused by a urinary tract infection; on the other hand, there is no good evidence to suggest that the use of cervical traction, manipulation or collar (process) is any better than placebo in altering the effects (outcome) of cervical spondylosis.

The term 'intermediate outcome' is used to describe measures that lie between true process and definitive outcome. The value of intermediate outcomes is that they are easier to measure, yet they predict (or are assumed to predict) definitive outcome. For example, the immunization rate is the sum of each injection given (process), which is easy to measure, yet it has an excellent predictive value because it is known that a high immunization rate will prevent or severely restrict (outcome) the diseases against which protection is being given. Thus, the immunization rate can be used as a proxy for a definitive outcome. In this situation it is unnecessary to wait what could be years for definitive measures of outcome, such as the number of cases of infection that ultimately occur in the immunized population, and the deaths or permanent disability that might result.

Audits of structure, process and outcome

Donabedian's framework for assessing quality defines one of the major parameters for describing audit. Thus, an audit of structure indicates an audit designed principally to assess the quality of the environment in which care is provided. A process audit describes the quality of work done by health professionals, and an audit of outcome will assess the benefits achieved for patients. It is possible to design an audit that will assess all three aspects of quality. However, audits that assess the performance of the individual clinician or the practice team, which is what people are primarily interested in, will investigate a combination of process and outcome. Several of the case studies illustrate audits of process and intermediate outcome.

Summary

This chapter has defined audit and described three characteristics of quality care: structure, process and outcome. The audit approach can be applied to any or all of these, using methods which are described in Chapters 7 and 8.

4   Who does audit?

AUDIT can be performed by individuals (doctor, nurse or other health professional) or by a practice team investigating its own care. This is known as internal audit. Equally, there can be an audit of peers or an audit carried out by others external to the health professionals concerned (*see* Box 4.1).

Box 4.1: Types of audit

- Internal audit
  - individual(s)
  - practice team.
- Peer audit.
- External audit.

Internal audit

The term 'internal audit' is self-explanatory. Internal audit is controlled and carried out by those whose own performance is to be assessed. As was said in the previous chapter, it is in the nature of professional people that they should regularly question their own work and justify their actions, both to themselves and to the outside world. In the context of general practice, internal audit helps individuals and practice teams to carry out their implied or stated intentions, and to determine whether to change their behaviour, i.e. their way of practising.

Regular internal audit can be difficult to sustain, often because other activities in a practice may claim priority. Owing to the immediate demands of patient care, and those of running the practice, audit may be an exercise for which the practice team will not have time; audit may be performed only when there is an enthusiast in the practice who will organize it and carry it out, invariably on a subject of his or her own choice. It is only if a practice team decides that the benefits of internal audit (*see* Chapter 2) are important or necessary, that resources – time, space, money, skills – will be allocated to it regularly.

Internal audit is fundamental to good care. However, its main advantages and disadvantages are related to the fact that it is private within a practice. As an advantage, it offers the opportunity for frank discussion, especially where things have gone wrong or where resulting changes may be disturbing for some members. As a disadvantage, it is easy for team members to collude and avoid awkward questions, looking instead at areas that seem safe.

Peer audit

One's peers are those who are equal to one in any stated respect. In the context of audit in medicine, the word applies to a person in the same specialty or branch of medicine who has comparable experience and training. All principals in general practice are regarded as peers; registrars in training, despite being doctors working in general practice, constitute a separate peer group.

When medical audit was first introduced in the USA in the 1930s, it was based on the principle of a review carried out by a doctor's peers. 'It takes one to know one' was the thinking behind this approach. In British general practice, peer review was introduced through vocational training. Today, it is usual for groups of trainees to meet to review case notes together. Trainer workshops operate on the peer principle when reviewing performance (*see* Example 4.1), and the national and regional structure and arrangements for selecting and reselecting trainers are based on the principles of peer review. Peer groups in general practice tend to be local and concerned with items of mutual interest to members.

Example 4.1

The first trainer audit group in the Northern Region, which was set up in 1975, attempted to set criteria and standards for the care of patients with hypertension, enuresis and urinary tract infections. Two members of the group also scrutinized the records of each of the trainer's patients who died; selected cases were later discussed by the group. In addition, the group paid particular attention to the standard of their clinical record-keeping, especially as their first audit of a selected sample of records had shown how wide the gap was between intention and reality.

Source: Ashton *et al.* (1976)[1]

Local peer groups are ideal for generating interpractice criteria and standards. For example, in the mid-1980s most Northern Region trainers took part in peer group standard setting for common childhood conditions.[2,3] Similarly, peer groups of general practitioners in The Netherlands[4,5] have met to consider criteria and standards that had already been formulated by experts. Both approaches have their place in audit by peer review in general practice.

One of the strengths of peer audit is that it is performed by colleagues in the same field of medicine: in many respects, it is general practitioners who are best placed to understand the possibilities and limitations of their discipline. Peer audit, therefore, is likely to be appropriate in context, and, as such, acceptable to colleagues.

The main criticism of peer review is that it may become collusive. It is common for peers to recognize their own shortcomings in clinical practice when faced with the limitations of others during audit. For example, most practitioners are familiar with situations such as not writing up the case notes of patients seen at home, or prescribing penicillin indiscriminately for all sore throats. Because all practices are guilty of such shortfalls from time to time, especially when under pressure, they may not be examined as rigorously as possible and hence go uncorrected.

External audit

The key difference between external and internal audit is that in external audit the auditors do not have their own performance assessed. The auditors may be general practitioners from another part of the country, they may belong to another specialty or profession, or they may be lay people. Consequently, an external audit group may represent quite different interests, values and priorities from those of the health professionals being assessed.

External audit is threatening because it introduces assessors who are relatively detached and who can therefore be objective. External audit is often associated with health service management, but has its roots firmly in the medical profession (*see* Examples 4.2 and 4.3). In general practice, the best-known example of external review embodying external audit is the system operated jointly by the regional postgraduate organizations and the Joint Committee on Postgraduate Training for General Practice (JCPTGP), to set and monitor standards for vocational training, particularly for teaching practices. These external audits have an educational element, but their main purpose is regulatory, to ensure that training practices deliver the quality of service that they have been contracted to, so that registrars obtain the maximum benefit from their training experience.

Example 4.2

The earliest and best-known examples of external audit in the UK were the confidential enquiries into maternal and perinatal deaths carried out jointly by the Royal College of Obstetricians and Gynaecologists (RCOG) and epidemiologists. These audits involved a meticulous examination of the case notes of all women and infants who died; from these national data, risk factors were identified which led to changes in clinical practices. As a consequence, maternal mortality and perinatal mortality rates have fallen. Outcome has been improved.

Source: HMSO 1957[6] and 1960[7]

Example 4.3

More recently, the Royal College of Surgeons (RCS) and the Faculty of Anaesthetists have been examining perioperative deaths on a confidential basis. These enquiries have already pinpointed aspects of surgical practice which in some units are causing unnecessary morbidity or death.

Source: Campling et al. (1995)[8]

The MAAGs (Medical Audit Advisory Groups) function in a similar manner in relation to district health authorities (DHA) and family practitioner services, partly by stimulating and helping practices to implement internal and peer audit, and partly by carrying out external comparative audits in local practices and across the boundary with secondary care. Examples of such audits include H_2 blocker administration, risk-factor advice following coronary artery bypass, and the content of discharge letters.[9]

External audit, because it brings greater objectivity to the assessment of performance, is the prime means by which any practice's performance can be monitored against national or regionally agreed standards. It offers the best opportunity of raising basic standards, and of identifying individual practices and health professionals who fall below the minimum. The disadvantages are that because it can be seen as threatening, it tends to provoke a defensive attitude from those whose performance is being assessed. Doctors may be tempted to find out what the minimum standard is and simply comply with it, without realizing their full potential.

Multidisciplinary audit

Audit of patient care began as a single-profession activity – hence, for example, 'medical audit' or 'nursing audit'. In the early 1990s the term 'clinical audit' came into general use, recognizing that most subjects for audit embraced a multidisciplinary team of health professionals. Multidisciplinary clinical audit involving practice teams may be both internal and external.

Multidisciplinary audit may also be multisectoral, that is, spanning more than one sector of care. The interface between primary and secondary care is the most common example.

Multidisciplinary audit may also extend to the patient – so-called patient-focused audit. Although sound in principle, it is proving difficult to establish in practice.

A combination

Experience suggests that all three main forms of audit are desirable in judicious combination. Internal audit should be the foundation of any system of quality assurance that undergoes regular improvement. The practice team motivated to question and initiate change regularly and systematically from within is most likely to provide the best care, and to achieve the highest standards.

Local peer review is cheap, easy to organize, and can act as a source of new ideas. It is now accepted as a valuable educational method in general practice that can bring measured objectivity without being overthreatening.

External review is becoming more and more important, especially in establishing adherence to minimum standards. Practices tend to make sure that they function well if they know there is to be an external audit, especially if incentives or sanctions are attached. Holding on to teaching contracts is one example. Comparative audits of prescribing using PACT data is another.

It seems clear that the more a practice does to set and monitor its own standards, the less likely it is to be at risk from external review.

5 How to do it: getting started

THERE are two important steps to be taken when considering an audit:

1 Choosing the subject.
2 Working out a design most likely to achieve the desired objective.

Choosing a subject

It can be surprisingly difficult to decide on a topic for audit. Some basic ground rules that can be used to help are shown in Box 5.1: these should always be considered before committing resources.

Box 5.1: Ground rules for choosing an audit subject

Any subject chosen for audit should be seen by the practice team as:

- likely to benefit patients
- likely to benefit the practice
- relevant to professional practice
- relevant to professional development
- significant or serious in terms of the process and outcomes of patient care
- having the potential for improvement
- capable of holding the interest and involvement of team members
- likely to repay the investment of time, money and effort involved.

Following these guiding principles will ensure that the subject chosen is meaningful to those professionals whose care is being audited.

Audit is often challenging; some members of the practice may have misgivings about their involvement in the process. For those who are unsure of the value of audit, the least that is required is a demonstration of the benefits (described in Chapter 2), and the chosen subject should be relevant. For practices in the early stages of learning about audit, careful attention to the choice will pay dividends in the form of involvement, if not commitment, from colleagues who may have a healthy scepticism towards this major shift in general practice.

Sources of ideas

The most obvious way of identifying a subject is through the trigger of a significant or adverse event in a practice, for example, a patient complaint about treatment, as illustrated in Case study 11, or the premature death of a patient from a treatable cause, such as acute asthma, meningitis or hypertension, as in Case study 7.

Topics may arise as a result of a regular review, either within or from outside the practice. Thus, practices who collect routine statistics might identify problems relating to prolonged waiting times for appointments, the failure of certain patients with diabetes to attend for reviews, as in Case studies 12 and 15, or an immunization programme (see Case studies 5 and 14). Similarly, questions that need to be explored further may arise as a consequence of an external review, for example when a peer group reviews the practice following an MAAG visit, or after a review of a teaching practice by the regional education committee for general practice.

Another source is the individual in a practice who has a particular idea that he or she wishes to pursue (see Case study 13). Most audits in general practice start in this way. These individuals will have particular priorities, which take precedence over other issues. Some of these ideas make a valuable place to start, although the 'bee in the bonnet' syndrome can be a diversion. Audit topics do have to be relevant to other team members.

Making the selection

There are several different sources of ideas for audit which need to be brought together in the practice. A practice that has a philosophy of questioning and justifying is likely also to have the sort of approach to management described in Chapter 10, which is based on planning ahead and on documenting wherever possible where it stands at present. Such practices are likely to have some arrangement for prioritizing activities, including the selection of subjects for audit.

The selection of a topic for audit is likely to be made by the partners or the team in the context of a practice's overall development plan. It is important that the team has some criteria for making a rational choice. The general principles described in Box 5.1 provide a useful guide. Baker and Presley (1990)[1] list a series of questions that can also be applied (Box 5.2).

It is desirable that one member of the practice team should assume responsibility for keeping the candidate subjects for audit under review, otherwise topics will be forgotten or the process of choice will become haphazard. It is a function of practice management to assign such responsibility.

Box 5.2: Questions to consider when choosing priorities

- Is the problem common?
- Does it affect patient care?
- Does it have serious consequences in terms of morbidity or mortality?
- Can it be solved using audit?
- Is it a management problem, rather than one of audit?
- Is it a district health authority problem, rather than a practice problem?
- Would correcting the problem save more money than ignoring it?
- Does the team have the skill to perform the audit?
- Does the team feel motivated to tackle the problem?

Source: Baker and Presley, 1990[1]

Planning an audit

When setting out along the audit route it is often unclear quite what the process will be, or what methods are to be used and what resources are required. Unless considerable thought is given to these issues, it is quite possible to be precipitated into a data collection exercise only to discover, too late, that insufficient attention to the basic design casts doubt at a later stage on the validity of the project. It is not uncommon to find data being collected (often more than are needed for the purpose) that will not provide an answer to the question(s) being asked, or which are incompatible with data from other practices against which comparisons are to be made.

Failures in the execution of an audit demoralize the auditor, diminish the confidence of other team members whose care is being audited, and waste resources.

The key lies in thorough planning. Just as the practice as a whole is more likely to succeed if it identifies clearly where it wants to go and how to get there – the link with practice management again – so an audit is most likely to succeed if the same steps are followed. The most important of these are summarized in Box 5.3.

Box 5.3: Planning an audit: 10 guidelines

1 Define the nature of the perceived problem.
2 Produce a clear written statement of aims.
3 Select the most appropriate methods.
4 Decide upon other basic design features.

5 Identify the main analysis to be made.
6 State who the audit will involve.
7 Start small.
8 Have a short timescale.
9 Proceed step by step.
10 Indicate how the possible need for change is to be handled.

1 **Defining the problem.** A general statement on the subject for audit should be followed by further definition of the perceived problem. Case study 1 shows the value of this. For example, if the problem is one of managing asthma in children, the next question might focus on a specific aspect, such as early diagnosis, care during acute attacks, parental information or preventive therapy. Further definition is important, for both deciding the aims and choosing the methods.

2 **Statement of aims.** It is worth spending time reaching agreement in the practice on written aims which are unambiguous and capable of being tested. The process of refining the aims will be facilitated by the discussion, in particular the attempts to explain what the audit is about and what it should accomplish.

3 **Choosing the method.** Once the aims are clear, the method can be chosen. The choice will be influenced partly by appropriateness and partly by the availability of relevant resources. Chapter 7 gives details of the methods available.

4 **Design decisions.** It is important to decide whether the audit is to be confined to the practice, or whether others should be involved in some way, and if so what the consequences will be. The design may include provision for an intervention to be tested; in this case, data should be collected before and after the intervention so that change can be measured. Questions as to whether the audit should be retrospective or prospective, or whether sampling should be employed, are important and discussed in greater detail below.

Retrospective and prospective audits. Retrospective audits have the advantage that they can provide information quickly about the nature of care that has been given in the immediate past. Their weakness is that they are wholly dependent on the completeness of the clinical notes kept in the patient's record, and practitioners do not make clinical notes with the needs of some future auditor in mind. Retrospective clinical audits are better suited to the examination of the care of patients with chronic illness than for those who have acute problems, because key events in the progress of a chronic condition are more likely to have been recorded.

Prospective audits look forward and are planned, with the aim of collecting data in a particular manner. Their strength is that the data collected are likely to give an accurate picture of the care the auditor wants to describe, provided that the method of data collection has been designed appropriately. One disadvantage of prospective audits is that they can alert the clinicians, whose performance is to be audited, to be on the lookout for what is expected of them and so alter their behaviour, which in unaudited circumstances might have been different.

Another variant is the audit that provides a 'snapshot' of the practice at a given point in time. Like other audits, this provides an opportunity to determine whether pre-existing criteria and standards are being adhered to, or to provoke further exploration.

Sampling. The technique of sampling enables the auditor to limit the amount of data collected without diminishing their value, especially their representativeness. Provided that the minimum number of cases to be examined during the audit is known, and also the number of cases seen during the audit period, it is possible to make the best use of time by collecting data on only a proportion of cases.

Such an approach depends upon the study area, the number of cases presenting and the time over which data are to be collected. In a large practice with 200–300 known cases of diabetes, for example, it may not be necessary to capture data on every case to answer the questions asked. By choosing to audit only a proportion of those cases, valid answers may still be reached and time and effort saved. Sampling is simple provided that the whole population from which the sample is drawn can be identified. The care of diabetes is a good example (*see* Example 5.1).

Example 5.1

A practice wished to collect information about the compliance of diabetic patients with dietary advice, following a drive in the practice to improve this. The first step was to decide how many patient records should be examined to ensure representativeness. This was calculated to be 70 of a total population of 200 patients with diabetes (who were numbered). The second step was to generate a random set of numbers between 1 and 200 until 70 cases had been identified.

Random samples used to be drawn using random number tables – the more romantic enthusiasts then used such devices as the DoH lottery number generator. Today the random number function on any calculator suitable for GCSE mathematics is the nearest source to hand.

This method is appropriate for general practice audit: the cases identified probably represent a spectrum of the diabetic illness within the practice.

A simpler method, known as systematic sampling, involves choosing a proportion of cases, for example 10% by identifying every 10th case on a register; the first case is chosen at random, for instance, number 7 on the register; the next case is 17, then 27, and so on. However, a filing system in which patients are grouped by address can introduce bias into this sampling method.

Practices that require a more sophisticated approach to sampling are advised to consult a statistician at the DHA or specialists in the local Department of Public Health. There is also an excellent chapter by Russell and Russell (1990)[2] which describes statistical analysis for audit in general practice.

5 **Analysis.** As part of the design of the audit it often helps to decide upon the main analyses to be made, and even to rough out the shape further by drawing up draft tables. The purpose is not to anticipate the results, but to generate an appropriate design. In larger audits this process might involve the use of a pilot to test the proposed design and method.

6 **Who is involved?** In a subject as sensitive as audit it is important to write down who is to be involved, to ensure that everyone is aware and can make the appropriate commitment. This active participation should also ensure commitment to any of the changes found to be necessary after audit.

7–9 **Step by step.** The principles of starting small and proceeding step by step over a short timescale are virtually self-evident. They set clear limits within which the audit takes place. These points need emphasizing because many auditors are easily carried away by their own enthusiasm.

10 **Managing change.** It is useful to have some idea about how the results are to be managed, especially if difficulties are expected: for example, the results could be critical of a particular individual. The ease with which this stage is handled will depend to a large extent on the professionalism of the practice's management systems (*see* Chapter 10).

The use of resources

It is important to decide on the maximum level of resources a practice team is prepared to commit to an audit. In doing this, it is also important to ensure that the subject examined is appropriate to the skills and resources available. Resources can be divided into time, money and people. Time is usually a limited resource: if staff are undertaking an audit, they are probably not able to perform another activity – known in economics as an opportunity cost. Although money can be used to buy more time, there is also an opportunity cost associated with this strategy. The original decision need not be rigid, and it is almost inevitable that the required resources will be underestimated. Nevertheless, an initial estimate of the available resources may help to determine the choices for such potentially expensive items as data collection.

The successful planning of an audit also includes continuous review. As each step of the audit becomes clear, the resources being used should be reassessed and compared with the original estimates, to ensure that the aims can be achieved. Regular checks are especially important if a practice team is performing more than one audit at a time, or if the ongoing audit is part of regular performance monitoring. Audit has to be efficient and effective, to give value for money, and to contribute to the practice's overall purpose; it should not become an end in itself.

Summary

The emphasis in this chapter has been on the need for a planned approach to audit. Success is more likely if early attention is given to aims that can be achieved using the resources available.

6 How to do it: criteria, standards and clinical guidelines

THIS chapter describes the first step in the audit cycle (*see* Chapter 3), when the partners or the practice team identify their current criteria and standards for good patient care and define new ones. Considering criteria and standards at the planning stage of an audit helps to define its aims. Standard setting is not an easy subject. Nevertheless, it is important to understand the basic methods because practices which master these can think about any audit with confidence, and will have a much better feel for the principles underlying the construction of modern, clinical guidelines.

The first part of the chapter places criteria, standards and clinical guidelines in their clinical and operational context within the practice. A description of their most important features follows. The chapter concludes with practical suggestions about the process of developing criteria and standards within practices and peer groups, and of adapting national clinical guidelines to meet a practice's own requirements.

The context

Doctors in any field of medicine work from a basis of 'good practice'. Good practice is the received wisdom of the day, which indicates the best way of diagnosing or managing a patient's condition. It guides the decisions made by doctors about individual patients, and it is the yardstick against which a doctor's handling of a case may be judged, for example by colleagues carrying out a peer review or in a court of law.

In its broadest sense good practice is largely implicit. Implicit criteria and standards of good practice reflect the 'right' way of, for example, treating a sore throat or pain in the neck caused by cervical spondylosis, or handling a bereaved person. Some standards are very personal and subjective. Thus, for instance, the feeling of comfort in the waiting room, courtesy, kindliness, a caring attitude and consideration for the feelings of relatives are all important components of quality, yet are founded on the experience, expectations and values of individuals, especially those receiving care. The problem with implicit criteria and standards is that there is scope for misunderstanding and variation in their interpretation, because they are subjective or because the evidence supporting them is conflicting or limited. It is difficult to assess performance in an individual case against subjective, generally stated principles, and it is virtually impossible to make meaningful comparisons between groups of cases without explicit statements of expected performance.

This is why there is a growing trend in medicine to use explicit, objective, evidence-based written statements to describe clinically effective care where it is possible to do so. The value of this approach is that it encourages health professionals to think more critically about what should be accomplished – what good practice and good performance should actually be – and consequently about the value of measuring their performance against a given standard. Explicit, objective statements can be communicated easily to other team members, so that the chances of misunderstanding are reduced and individuals can find it easier to stick to what has been agreed. Explicit statements are also essential for valid comparisons of quality between practices.

The major disadvantage of explicit, objective statements is that there is a limit to what can actually be defined and measured in this way. The assessor may focus only on the measurable, and claim that only the measurable reflects quality. However, the attributes of care with implicit standards mentioned above are nevertheless part of good-quality care and have to be taken into account. Although explicit standards should be used wherever possible, an assessor should be prepared to make judgements on matters where standards can only be implicit.

And so to clinical guidelines. Clinical guidelines consist of aggregates of criteria and standards, brought together so that there is an authoritative statement on a clinical subject, for example the investigation and treatment of angina, the management of asthma in childhood, or low-back pain. The modern clinical guideline takes a great deal of money, effort and expertise to construct, not least because it must incorporate and be an accurate expression of the best of science at that point in time. Today, the quickest and easiest thing for a practice to do is to take a recognized national guideline and make its own modifications to it if it wishes. Guidelines need to be acceptable for everyday operational use.

So, a general practice today will have at its disposal two basic approaches to standard setting. It will be able to decide its own – absolutely essential when considering in-house, clinical and operational protocols specifically designed for internal use. Second, it may draw on the growing library of national clinical guidelines which can be taken off the shelf, modified for local use if necessary, and then put into action. More and more practices are doing this, because it is easy and saves time by not 'reinventing the wheel'. Whatever the route chosen, these criteria, standards and clinical guidelines need to be 'owned' by the practice because they are the template against which the performance of individual clinicians or the team will be assessed through audit. Ownership carries with it a far greater chance of commitment to adhere to the desired standards in the ups and downs of everyday practice.

Examples of practices working with simple, explicit statements are given in Case studies 4 and 15. In Case studies 7 and 14, practice teams are trying to develop them. The audit cycle described in Chapter 3 begins with the stage of defining explicit statements describing criteria and standards for care. In Chapter 10 this process is directly related to that stage in the management cycle at which a practice team starts by defining its aims, objectives of standards for care. It is therefore helpful to see in more detail what is meant by criteria, standards and clinical guidelines, and in particular how they can be developed.

Criteria and standards

The term *criterion* is used to describe a definable and measurable item that describes quality, and which can be used to assess it. Criteria are usually written in the form of statements describing what should happen (*see* Example 6.1).

Example 6.1: Single statement criteria

- Females of susceptible age should be immunized against rubella.
- All children requesting attention for acute problems will be seen on the same day.
- Any patient will normally be offered a non-urgent appointment with any doctor within 48 hours, except in an epidemic.

A *standard* describes the level of care to be achieved for any particular criterion; continuing with the example of rubella immunization in Example 6.1, the standard might specify that 98% of the female population at risk should receive protection. The full criterion and standard are given in Example 6.2.

Example 6.2

- Females of susceptible age should be immunized against rubella (*criterion*).
- 98% of all females of susceptible age will be immunized against rubella (*standard*).

It may take practice to be able to make the distinction between criteria and standards. The best way to learn is to write out some simple statements similar to those illustrated in Examples 6.1 and 6.2.

There are many opportunities for using single-statement criteria and standards of the kind illustrated above, in isolation. However, it is possible, through the careful selection of criteria, to build up a picture or map of the most important characteristics of a disease or a symptom and of best practice in terms of investigation, treatment, and overall management. These aggregated criteria and standards describing good care are the basis of clinical guidelines (of which more later) and of internal protocols defining practice-specific procedures.

Clinical guidelines and protocols can be presented as a series of statements or displayed in the form of a flowchart, known as an algorithm. Both are used today. The algorithm shows the branched decision-making process and its options at each stage. Figs 6.1 and 6.2 are extracts from clinical algorithms used in general practice for the management of constipation and acute diarrhoea in children.[1] Further information about the construction and use of clinical algorithms in primary care is contained in

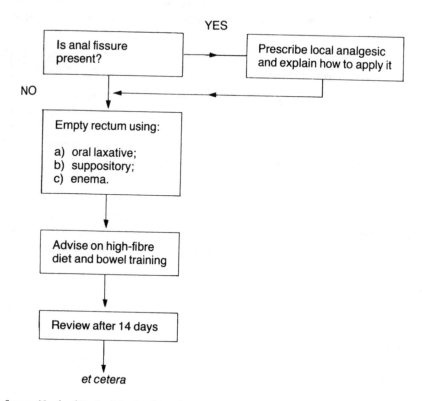

Source: North of England Study of Standards and Performance in General Practice (1990)[1]

Figure 6.1 An extract from the branching algorithm for management of constipation in children

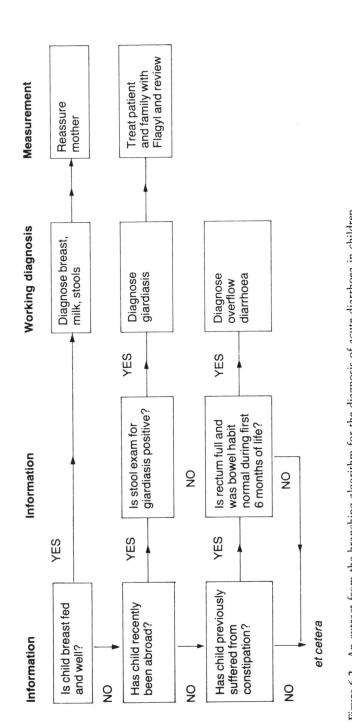

Figure 6.2 An extract from the branching algorithm for the diagnosis of acute diarrhoea in children

	Criterion	Standard
Structure	Patient records will include summary cards.	Should apply to 50% of records.
Process	All patients aged 20–65 years will have their blood pressure recorded in the notes at least once, within the last five years.	This should apply to: 50% of records in year 1, 75% of records in year 2, 95% of records in year 3, following the introduction of the standard.
Outcome	Patients with established hypertension aged 20–35 years will have a diastolic level less than 90 mmHg within the first year of treatment.	The target level will be achieved in 80% of cases.

Figure 6.3   Examples of criteria and standards

the excellent paper by Schoenbaum and Gottlieb (1990)[2] and in the British Medical Journal series[3] of clinical algorithms.

Content of criteria and standards

Criteria and standards can be further defined by the particular characteristic of care – structure, process or outcome – they are describing (*see* Fig. 6.3 for examples).

Structural criteria and standards define aspects of the environment for care. An example of a structural criterion indicating quality would be the statement: 'Patient record cards should contain a summary card'.

Continuing with this example, the structural standard, indicating the level to be achieved, might be set at 50% initially; it could be raised as practice teams reach this minimum standard, to ensure that improvement is maintained.

Process criteria and standards describe the care provided for the patient. A process criterion might state, for example, that: 'The blood pressure of all patients aged 20–65 years should be taken and recorded at least once every five years'.

Continuing with this example, a process standard would specify the frequency with which the criterion should be achieved, for instance in the first, second and third years following the introduction of this particular criterion.

Criteria and standards of outcome describe the effects of care on the patient. Continuing with the example about blood pressure, an outcome criterion might state that: 'In young adult patients with hypertension a diastolic pressure of 90 mmHg or less should be achieved within one year of commencing treatment'.

The standard of outcome might require that 80% of such patients should achieve the criterion within the stated period.

In distinguishing between *process criteria and standards* and *criteria and standards of outcome*, it is important to remember that *process criteria* describe the care given and *outcome criteria* describe the effects on the patient. Better process does not always result in better outcome. For example, a practice team could pay assiduous attention to the process criteria and standards for blood pressure described above, making sure that blood pressure was measured and recorded in the notes to the standard required, and might be tempted to conclude that the patients were benefiting from this carefully regulated care. In fact, patients would benefit only if the practice team was able to show that the blood pressure level was controlled satisfactorily in accordance with the standard of outcome set. Were that not the case the only evidence of quality would be the frequency with which blood pressure measurements appeared in the notes. This distinction is nicely illustrated in Case study 15.

Level of standards

There is always controversy when decisions have to be made about the precise level at which a standard should be pitched. There are three options, all of which can be illustrated using current standards for mumps, measles and rubella (MMR) immunization in children under the age of two years.

A *minimum* standard describes the lowest acceptable standard of performance. Minimum standards are often used to distinguish between acceptable and unacceptable practice. For example, the DoH has defined its minimum standard for immunization in the New Contract as at least 70% of all children eligible. The DoH underlines the use of this standard to define what it considers to be the boundary between acceptable and unacceptable practice by not making a bonus payment for any immunization programme that fails to reach the 70% target.

An *ideal* standard describes the care it should be possible to give under ideal conditions, when there are no constraints on resources of any kind. An ideal standard, almost by definition, cannot be attained. Continuing with the example, an ideal standard would require that *all* children within a practice would have completed a course of immunization by two years.

An *optimum* standard lies between the minimum and the ideal. Setting an optimum standard requires a judgement to be made about the best balance between, for example, the outcome for the individual patient and equity for patients as a whole in terms of resources available. Optimum standards represent the standard of care most likely to be achieved under the normal conditions of practice. They are most likely to reflect the good practice any conscientious general practitioner could be expected to achieve. The DoH definition of the 'optimum' standard for childhood immunization is a 90% immunization rate of those eligible. To reinforce the attainment of this standard, the DoH gives a higher payment for all practice immunization programmes that reach or exceed the optimum standard.

The derivation of criteria and standards

Criteria and standards can be derived from either the most recent medical literature and the best experience of clinical practice, or from current societal and professional values – 'normative' criteria. Criteria can also reflect patterns of care taken from existing data and thereby current practice – 'empirical' criteria. In some ways empirical standards are weaker than those drawn from the 'state of the art', precisely because they are a reflection of statistical averages that might or might not reflect good care.

For a practice considering defining criteria and standards for the first time, a combination of the two is best. It is worthwhile taking current patterns of care into account, but these should be set in the context of what it is best to do in terms either of the science of medicine or of the values of society and the health professions.

Internal and external standards

Another way of looking at criteria and standards is to consider who sets them. There are two options, internal or external. Internal criteria and standards, most often displayed as operational protocols, are determined and set by practitioners whose care is subsequently assessed by audit. In effect, the individual practitioner, the practice team (comparable to self-audit) or possibly the local peer group sets the criteria. The advantage of internally determined protocols is ownership: health professionals who have created their own are better motivated to implement the product of their own work because they decided that the need was there in the first place.

External criteria and standards are created by any individual or group who is not being assessed. The advantage of externally generated criteria and standards is that they are likely to be more rigorous in their construction. The disadvantage is that they may be imposed; if so, those whose care is to be assessed may question them and be grudging in their willingness to implement and maintain them.

The solution lies in a balance between internal and external criteria and standards. A practice team should construct and use its own internal protocols for everyday practice wherever possible, so that its members can see what they are trying to do and what they actually achieve. National external standards, usually expressed as clinical guidelines, should be used selectively: few areas in medicine as yet lend themselves to dogmatic statements that cannot be challenged.

Working on criteria and standards

There are several points that should be borne in mind when constructing criteria and standards which are to be used for audit. In particular, it is necessary to:

- make unambiguous statements
- keep the task focused on the topic
- refer to the literature indicating current practice
- choose criteria and standards in line with current practice
- ensure that criteria and standards are based on fact.

Health professionals often fail to take account of the work of others. Referring to published work is essential to avoid the danger of making statements that are inaccurate. The librarian at a local postgraduate centre can provide invaluable help in identifying references, and a growing number of practices have direct access to the international literature of medicine through CD-ROM and the Internet.

It is often best to decide criteria and standards in a group because the testing of ideas by people working together is likely to achieve a more robust result than can be attained by individuals working in isolation. Experience suggests that there are three specific factors that will facilitate the work of a group and thereby improve its chances of success:

1 At least one member of the group should be thoroughly familiar with current practice. An expert may be invited to attend the group so that he or she can act as a clinical resource when necessary.

2 One member of the group should have had at least some experience in the technique of writing criteria and standards, and of translating these into workable protocols in a format most acceptable to the practice.

3 The group should have a competent chairman. It is often difficult to be productive and achieve a consensus about what should be done, and a

good chairman will help the group to get a good result, whereas a leaderless group will get lost.

Clinical guidelines

Clinical guidelines are 'systematically developed statements to assist practitioner and patient decisions about appropriate health care for specific clinical circumstances'.[4]

Clinical guidelines should 'identify recommendations for the appropriate and cost-effective management of clinical conditions and the appropriate use of clinical procedures with the principal aim of promoting good performance'.[5]

Clinical guidelines may be used for a number of purposes, including:[4]

- assisting clinical decision making by patients and practitioners
- educating individuals or groups
- assessing and assuring the quality of care
- guiding the allocation of measures for health care
- reducing the risk of legal liability for negligent care.

The properties of effective clinical guidelines have been summarized by Grimshaw and Russell[6] (Box 6.1).

Box 6.1: Properties of effective guidelines

Attribute	Explanation
Validity	Guidelines are valid if, when followed, they lead to the health gains and costs predicted for them.
Reproducibility	Guidelines are reproducible if, given the same evidence on methods of guideline development, another guideline produces essentially the same recommendations.
Reliability	Guidelines are reliable if, given the same clinical circumstances, another health professional interprets and applies them in essentially the same way.
Representative development	Guidelines should be developed by a process that entails participation by key affected groups.
Clinical applicability	Guidelines should apply to patient populations defined in accordance with scientific evidence of best clinical judgement.
Clinical flexibility	Guidelines should identify exceptions to their recommendations and indicate how patient preferences are to be incorporated in decision making.

Clarity	Guidelines must use unambiguous language, precise definitions, and user-friendly formats.
Meticulous documentation	Guidelines must record participants involved, assumptions made, and evidence and methods used.
Scheduled review	Guidelines must state when and how they are to be reviewed (under two separate circumstances – the identification or not of new scientific evidence as professional consensus).

Adapted by Grimshaw and Russell from *Guidelines for Practice from Development to Use* National Academy of Sciences (1992). Courtesy of National Academy Press, Washington DC.

The properties of a modern clinical guideline as set out in Box 6.1 show only too well that, although such guidelines are founded on the basic criteria and standards described earlier, they require resources that are beyond the average practice; hence the trend to national clinical guidelines. The various aspects of their use have been described comprehensively by the RCGP in a recent statement.[7]

More clinical guidelines of special relevance to general practice are now becoming available, and can be used as the basis for audit where a practice deems this appropriate. For example, the North of England evidence-based development project has produced guidelines for the primary care management of two common conditions, namely asthma in adults[8] and stable angina.[9] The Royal College of General Practitioners has just published an evidence-based guideline on low back pain,[10] and general practitioners in Scotland are involved in the Scottish Intercollegiate Guidelines Network (SIGN)[11] which has produced recent guidelines[12] on, for instance, the prevention of visual impairment in diabetic patients, immediate discharge and *Helicobacter pylori*: eradication therapy in dyspeptic disease.

The adoption and use of existing evidence-based clinical guidelines holds the promise of bringing the fruits of research quickly into general practice. Audit based on such guidelines should show a practice and the outside world how effective it is in translating ideals into reality.

Summary

Once the basic technique for constructing criteria and standards has been learned and mastered, health professionals will find this activity stimulating and rewarding. If criteria and standards have developed within a practice, much will be learnt about what the members of that practice want: it is a valuable team-building exercise as well as a learning exercise. By concentrating on explicit criteria and standards wherever possible, a practice team will develop a series of statements about patient care which it considers to be important and which reflects quality. This can then be used as the basis for subsequent audit or performance monitoring. Such statements can be revised and updated regularly.

7 How to do it: data and methods I

THIS chapter describes the principal sources of data for audit in general practice. On occasion, data sources, data collection and audit methods can be considered to be equivalent, for example in surveys and interviews. In other cases, such as medical records, the data may be used for more than one audit purpose, i.e. as more than one data source. For simplicity, the methods for carrying out an audit that use more than one data source are described in Chapter 8.

Many practices now have computers and use them for both data storage and audit. This can make audit easier, particularly when dealing with larger amounts of data. However, much audit can be done with simple data collection and analysis using manual methods.

Many audits start with data collection, and the first stage of the audit cycle, i.e. defining criteria and standards, is omitted. This is legitimate, especially if the purpose of the audit is to carry out a preliminary reconnaissance of some aspects of a practice team's work.

The eight most commonly used sources of data are shown in Box 7.1. Each data source will be described using a format that indicates the origin of the data, how they can be collected and used, and an assessment of their strengths and weaknesses.

Box 7.1: Data sources and data collection

- Routine practice data
- External data
- Medical records
- Practice activity analysis
- Prospective recording of specific data
- Surveys
- Interviews
- Direct observation

Routine practice data

Routine practice activity generates data that are often used for regular performance monitoring. These data are varied and may be quite detailed.

Source

Data that should be readily available are the records of practice claims to the DHA. For example, every practice should have a record of immunizations carried out, cervical cytology examinations undertaken, hospital referrals made, prescribing patterns (PACT), and night calls made between 10 pm and 8 am.

Many practices routinely keep other data to describe workload. For example, appointments and visiting books will show the number of patients consulting, the number of house calls made, the number of out-of-hours calls, the attendances at antenatal clinics, and the number of patients seen in the treatment room by the practice nurse.

Every practice also has basic registration data that will indicate patients' age and sex, marital status and postcode. Some practices may have other registers, for example a disease index, registers of certain age groups – e.g. children under five or patients over 75 – or a register of the permanently housebound who live alone. Occupation may also be recorded. Many practices also keep a record of the annual number of livebirths, stillbirths and terminations, and every practice has either the death certificate books or hospital correspondence which, taken together, can give details of most of the patients who have died, together with a cause of death.

Finally, the annual practice accounts contain data under the main headings of expenditure and income, from which financial trends may be detected.

How to collect the data

The first step is to recognize the potential value of data that practice teams record routinely in support of their management functions. Second, the purpose of audit data collection must be clarified (for instance to indicate trends in immunization rates). These data should then be structured, so that the information is readily available and accessible. It is then a matter of assembling the data using a simply designed data collection sheet or entering them directly into the practice computer. Results can be analysed either manually or using a basic computer program such as EpiInfo (*see also* Chapter 9).

Uses

These data have four main uses:

1 Data may be used to control some practice activities. For example, a practice team intending to achieve the top target for immunization regularly will need to know who has been immunized, on a weekly basis. Case studies 2 and 5 show data being used in this way. Similarly,

routine monitoring is used to control aspects of income and expenditure to ensure that all claims are made and that cash flow is satisfactory.

2 Routine monitoring can alert a practice team to minor changes which, if allowed to continue over time, may become significant. For instance, an insidious increase in the interval that patients have to wait between requesting an appointment and being seen may be highlighted by routine monitoring, allowing remedial action to be taken before a crisis occurs and complaints are made.

3 Routine monitoring may chart the progress of a change in practice policy. For example, the impact of a practice decision to immunize all adults against tetanus can be monitored either through the number of prescriptions being claimed from the DHA in non-computerized practices, or from a practice's computer record.

4 Routinely collected data are used in several audit methods. For example, they should contribute to the overall profile of a practice which is built up during the course of a practice visit. In some practice activity analyses they can act as substitutes for or complements to data that have to be collected specifically for an audit, which are more expensive.

Strengths and weaknesses

The great strength of these data is that they are cheap and easy to collect, because they are derived from regular practice activity. If used to monitor performance, they have an additional value in that they can act as a trigger for more specific audits designed to explore certain aspects of performance in more detail. Their weakness is that they are limited in scope to a screening function and often contribute only marginally to other audits a practice may have in mind.

External data

As changes in the NHS have gathered pace, so too has the flood of data from external sources. Some of this will be information, i.e. data that has already been interpreted. More often, data will require analysis to transform it into information relevant to the context of general practice.

Source

The local DHA is becoming the most common source of external data, some of which may be the trigger for a practice audit. For example, the DHA is now the best source of data on a practice's prescribing patterns. The PACT analysis and feedback indicate what is possible. Similar analyses and feedback can shortly be expected on patterns of referral to hospitals.

DHAs are also becoming a source of non-routine data. For example, it is possible to request specific analyses of the age–sex and geographical distribution of the practice population. The DHA could also be asked to provide a breakdown of census data relating to the practice area. Local community trusts collect detailed data on the workload and case mix of community nurses and health visitors. These describe a major aspect of care given to patients in a practice, and are relevant to a practice team trying to build a picture of practice activity.

How to collect the data

The main problem with health authority information is volume. The only practical strategy for handling large volumes of data is for the practice, as part of its management functions, to designate one person in the team to be responsible for reviewing a particular subject area regularly, and for reporting on any matters of potential interest. The practice should also have a mechanism for bringing data from widely disparate sources together and to index them again as part of the practice's management systems. However, it may be possible to collaborate with the local DHA or the local audit group, in such a way as to limit the effort needed to access and use these valuable data.

Uses

The main benefit of data from external sources lies in their relevance to practice policy making and in stimulating new initiatives. For example, a significant change in the DHA quarterly returns on additions to or removals from the practice list may lead to a further audit designed to establish cause. Improved feedback on immunization rates, cervical cytology screening, breast cancer screening and the use of the X-ray and laboratory services by individual partners should stimulate regular discussions within the team, some of which may prompt a more detailed audit of some particular aspect. Detailed information of the type generated by PACT level 3 can provide the basis for a variety of future audits, as illustrated in Case study 6. For instance, the implementation of an agreed practice policy for prescribing antibiotics can be monitored through PACT data, with minimal effort for data collection but not for interpretation.

Strengths and weaknesses

As with the routine general practice data, the format of externally produced routine data is fixed and may not always be appropriate to the task.

However, they are usually cheap (sometimes free) and can provide comparisons with other practices. DHAs hold increasingly valuable data sets on health needs assessment. It is the responsibility of a practice team to find out what is available and make the best use of it.

Data from medical records

Medical records in general practice vary widely in their structure and content, and therefore in their usefulness as an audit tool. Some practices have well-ordered records which give a reasonably clear and complete account of the care given to patients, containing summaries of significant events, showing current medication, and recording the clinical details in a common format. However, records can be disorganized, with only a few clinical details recorded.

The medical record should be one of the most important sources of data, especially for retrospective clinical audit, because it is the account closest to direct observation and is a means of knowing what happened to any patient. However, the potential discrepancy between the case and the record will depend entirely on whether a practice has policies and standards for record-keeping that ensure a minimum content consistent with a coherent account of care given.

The introduction of the A4 record into general practice (not yet widespread, other than in Scotland) has improved the standard of record-keeping and thereby the potential value of medical records for retrospective audit. The A4 record, by virtue of its structure and size, encourages a more consistent recording of clinical events and the data, such as summaries, prescriptions and demographic details, are located in properly identified areas.

Computerized records provide a major opportunity to access data retrospectively because of the highly structured format of the record and the ability of an increasing number of computer programs to search for selected data items.

How to collect the data

Records must be searched and the relevant data abstracted from the mass of other material. For paper records this can be a tedious task, because one can never be sure that the data sought actually exist without trawling through each individual record. This is not too difficult when only 20–30 records are involved, but it becomes substantial and time-consuming if 200–300 are to be examined. Moreover, the data required may be held in different parts of the record – in the correspondence or on the summary sheet, for instance.

To make abstraction as simple as possible, clinical records should be well structured. It is particularly helpful if a common format is agreed among the practice team. The problem-orientated approach is one way; a useful variation of this is to use the following headings:

- Presumptive diagnosis
- Evidence for diagnosis
- Management decisions
- Reasons for management decisions.

It is equally essential to have a well-structured audit recording sheet, so that the data abstracted can be collected efficiently and accurately.

Data that have been computerized are *usually* easier to access than those from paper records, although some of the earlier software programs offered frustratingly limited opportunities from what should be a rich data source.

Uses

Retrospective data collected from records can provide insights into previous clinical practice; more accurately, they can give insights into the aspects of clinical care that have been recorded. In Case study 4, the patient record has been used in this way.

An examination of the patterns of previous care may indicate problems that require further explanation. It is usual to use a retrospective audit to identify a problem initially, which can be further examined using a prospective audit in which the clinicians are asked to record relevant data in a specifically structured, and therefore easily abstractable, form.

Strengths and weaknesses

The use of previously recorded data has the advantage of requiring only limited effort and it can be collected over a short timescale. The 'quality' of the results depends partly on the overall standard of the records. If the records are unstructured and handwritten, the return may not reflect the effort required. However, if an extensive data set has been collected, retrospective data collection should always be considered as one of the data sources for a practice audit.

Practice activity analysis

Practice activity analysis (PAA) is the term used to describe the examination of patterns of care in general practice, particularly those actions that doctors undertake frequently, such as prescribing, using laboratory and X-ray facilities, and referring patients to hospital. It was one of the earliest audit methods introduced into general practice, beginning in 1975 with the pioneering service provided by Drs Crombie and Fleming at the Birmingham Research Unit of the Royal College of General Practitioners.[1] Practice activity analysis is relatively easy to design and carry out. It quantifies the major activities in general practice and thereby helps to build a picture of the work of a practice. There are two principal types of practice activity analysis: one relates to the activities of a single practice team; the other follows the model of largescale data collection from several practices of the kind described by the College.

For the individual practice, practice activity analysis is a form of structured data collection which is clearly formatted for audit purposes. Largescale practice activity analysis involves contributions to a general pool of data to generate 'norms' against which any individual practice can be compared. Various national agencies provide this service, the best known being the RCGP Birmingham Research Unit. However, it is more likely that local audit groups (such as MAAGs or their successors) will provide a service which will enable local comparisons of activity data.

How to collect the data

A structured form is used to record a preselected set of data items (*see* Fig. 7.1). These can be analysed easily within the practice on a computer using a spreadsheet program or a database such as dBase III. Another option is to seek help from the DHA information services manager or public health department. Again, the local audit group should possess these skills.

Any member of the practice team can be involved in data collection – nursing and administrative staff are often more rigorous and accurate than doctors. Most often, however, the bulk of data collection will take place at the time of a consultation.

Uses

Practice activity analysis can provide an overview of important aspects of a practice's function, such as use of laboratory and X-ray facilities or workload patterns. Regular and planned events are particularly suitable for this mode of analysis. They can be used to monitor progress to previously agreed standards, or as the starting point for a more detailed audit of a particular aspect. The content of the data set needs to be defined with the required uses in mind: trawling randomly for chance events is unlikely to be efficient. Case studies 1, 5 and 10 show the use of practice activity analysis.

Patient characteristics		Case numbers								
		1	2	3	4	5	6	7	8	
Patient > 60 years	1									
Owns own house	2									
Married	1									
Family history of diabetes	3									
Smokes 10+/day	1									
Uses insulin	2									

Key:
1 = Yes; 2 = No; 3 = Don't know/no response.

Figure 7.1 Practice activity analysis coding sheet

Interpractice comparisons can provide an interesting perspective on a practice's performance, and may influence the process of care in such areas as immunization. Because they can provide comparisons with a selected data set, they can enable comparisons to be made of practices working in similar circumstances, or at least provide the information necessary to understand the reasons for any differences in those circumstances.

Strengths and weaknesses

Practice activity analysis has three major advantages:

1 It can provide a framework for identifying patterns of events which hitherto may have been hidden.
2 It furnishes direct comparisons with the performance of colleagues. Opportunities for external review, as part of peer review, may originate from this point.

3 It can be used as a prompt or trigger for more specific audits on areas of interest or concern.

Practice activity analysis has two possible weaknesses:

1 If there is a substantial commitment to data collection, which has to continue for a long time, the willingness of a practice team may evaporate and the accuracy of the data can be compromised.
2 Practice activity analysis is more suited to showing patterns and rates than it is for revealing the underlying reasons for such patterns. For example, although practice activity analysis of hospital referrals would disclose variations in patterns and rates, a specifically designed prospective audit would shed light on the decision-making processes of clinicians, which account substantially for such variations in the first place.

Prospective recording of specific data

Many audits require the collection of a specific data set, comprising a number of data items not usually recorded or which need to be recorded in a particular format. In these circumstances the data must be newly collected, either at a particular point in time – a cross-sectional study – or over a period of time – a longitudinal study. The definition of the items will have been refined through the process of planning the audit and formulating the clinical criteria and standards.

How to collect the data

One of the simplest methods of collecting specific data is to ask the health professional to record the required items at the appropriate time, for example when writing a prescription or making a referral, or ordering an investigation. However, the clinician needs guidance to ensure that only the required items are collected, because every item collected adds time and effort to the consultation. Wherever possible the items should be recorded on a computer, which will allow the rapid generation of aggregated data at the end of the collection period.

An alternative strategy is for the data collector to record the required items on audio tape, which can then be transcribed by a secretary on to a paper or computer record. This technique is particularly useful for data collection outside the surgery. The practice administrative staff might also collect some of the non-clinical material relevant to each case.

Uses

Audits of care for relatively frequent events are often well served by data set recording. Usually, these data relate to the process of care, i.e. the care provided by the professional during the consultation. An audit of prescribing patterns, for instance, which requires a data set of age, sex, presenting symptoms, working diagnosis, treatment and result, might necessitate the use of the prospective data collection method. Another example might be the planned monitoring of care for a particular group of patients who have a chronic condition, such as hypertension, asthma or recurrent urinary tract infection. An encounter form can be held in each patient's record for completion at the time of consultation. Case study 2 gives an example of this.

Strengths and weaknesses

Data collection forms act as a prompt for the doctor or nurse. This may, however, distort the results of the audit, which might not have been as positive if there had been no such prompt. This effect can be overcome only with considerable effort, and for the purpose of operational practice audit the resulting lack of distortion is generally not worth the expenditure of effort to avoid it. Indeed, it could be argued that this is a benefit, if the changes are made in patient care as well as in recording.

The minimum data set and recording system do require forethought, which can assist in clarifying the purpose of the audit. It is important to remember that a considerable amount of data can be collected by this method, not all of which can be used effectively.

Surveys

Many practices are only just discovering the value of the survey as a valuable means of gathering information about the health of the practice population or about their expectations of its services. Essentially, surveys are a method of collecting data about some aspect of a patient's life by means of a questionnaire. Whichever method of survey is chosen, it is important to recognize the rules of survey methodology, and the practice team wishing to explore this method further will find it helpful to consult Abrahamson.[2] Time spent with this lively and concise work will save considerable effort – and potential disappointment – later.

Source

Surveys can be undertaken by post or on forms handed out in the surgery waiting room. The forms can vary from a relatively unstructured format, in which the questions elicit a variety of written answers, to a highly structured format in which the respondent ticks boxes. Surveys can be carried out on small or large numbers of people, different methods being used for various purposes. Surveys can be used to collect data about the process of care, the care patients receive, or the outcomes of care, including patient satisfaction. An increasing number of standardized questionnaires are commercially available, although care must be taken over choice. Local audit groups often have a useful selection of questionnaires appropriate to general practice. Case study 3 demonstrates the use of a postal survey.

How to collect the data

Survey questionnaires are targeted at specific groups of people. The group may be identified by a particular characteristic, such as age or diabetes, or because they were engaged in a certain activity at a particular time, for example every woman who has attended an antenatal clinic in the past year, or every adult who has sat in the waiting room during the past month. The data can be used to perform a cross-sectional audit (that is, once only) or to review the process of care over time.

A record must be kept of who receives the questionnaire, when and why. The practice age–sex register (computer or card index) may be used to identify recipients. This information is vital to understand the response rates and the context in which the data were collected.

Uses

A wide range of audits can be supported by survey methodology. Provided that the questionnaire has been properly designed, information on issues such as the outcome of care for chronic disease, patient satisfaction or morbidity can be collected. The local public health department in the DHA may be a valuable source of advice.

Strengths and weaknesses

Surveys can produce a plethora of data unless appropriate thought has been give to data management and analysis. The use of sampling should always be considered to limit the data collected to what is sufficient to satisfy the audit design (*see* Chapter 5) but not excessive so as to be redundant. Surveys are also relatively costly in terms of production and postage (where necessary). If many people do not return the questionnaires, reminders will have to be sent. None of these hazards should dissuade a practice from considering surveys. Patients are often willing to provide information useful to their own health care or to improve the service they use, and surveys are a valuable way of achieving these ends.

Interviews

Data collected by interviewers is usually more detailed than survey data, although the number of respondents is usually limited. Despite the fact that much data collection in primary health care is based on a particular type of interview, i.e. the consultation, it is relatively uncommon for the data for a general practice audit to be collected in this manner. There may be several reasons for this.

1 Interviews should be carefully structured (even if they are 'unstructured').
2 It is recognized that analysis is sometimes difficult.
3 Interviewers are often expensive to employ, which substantially increases the costs of an audit.

Nevertheless, with careful attention to method, the selection of topics and techniques, interviews can prove to be a useful method of data collection for audit.

How to collect the data

The development of interview questionnaires and their analysis is well covered by Abrahamson.[2] A carefully worded questionnaire can elicit more detail about the health care and health status of an individual than any of the preceding methods. Although the answers may be translated into a coded form, the opportunity to select a certain feature and follow it through in depth is available. Additional comment can be recorded verbatim to illuminate the audit results – an important skill to be learned by those who use this method.

Uses

Complex or sensitive issues that cannot be addressed easily by methods such as postal questionnaires often lend themselves to investigation through interviews – for example, the effects of treatment, particularly if there are embarrassing side-effects, such as sexual dysfunction. Unusual or rare events may also be best investigated through the medium of the interview, e.g. the care provided for people who have a terminal illness, for which a sensitive approach is essential, or an audit of adverse events, such as preventable death in people under 65 years of age. Aspects of the process and outcomes of care can be examined using this technique.

Strengths and weaknesses

Interview technique is different from consultation techniques in general. Perhaps because of this doctors do not make the best interviewers. Some training in interview techniques is usually necessary to derive the most from this method. Consequently, it may be appropriate to 'buy in' the necessary interviewing and analysing skills.

The major advantage of this method is its potential to provide insights into complex issues.

Direct observation

There are several ways in which the process of care can be audited using direct observation, although it is one of the most difficult methods to use and analyse successfully. The most obvious technique is to have an observer in the consultation, although this invariably alters the dynamic being observed. Other techniques include the use of a 'one-way' mirror (now rather out of fashion) and audio and video recording. Some of these methods are regularly used for teaching in general practice, and have been advocated as a means of reviewing performance in the RCGP's *What sort of doctor?*.[3] All general practice registrars will have experience of video recording and analysis, and, in teaching practices at least, direct observation may become an increasingly used audit method.

How to collect the data

The capture of raw data is difficult in direct observation. Problems occur when the observations have to be reduced to reproducible data, because any implicit judgements made about the data hold as much value as implicit criteria and standards for care.

Several techniques exist for analysing the content of consultations, although all are time-consuming. If an audit has limited objectives, for example if the aim is to record whether a doctor gives advice on stopping smoking to a smoker with a chest infection, a relatively simple data collection form will suffice; unfortunately, a mass of raw data, in the form of consultations, might have to be reviewed in order to achieve even this limited objective.

Uses

The process of care, interpersonal skills and specific types of information exchange can all be examined using direct observation. However, this method has more value in education than in audit. For example, doctors who sit in on each other's consultations use this as an opportunity to learn from their colleagues' best practice. Video consultations are also discussed among peers, which is a less challenging approach to reviewing clinical performance in individual cases.

Strengths and weaknesses

Direct observation allows the doctor–patient interaction to be investigated. Its use as a method of examining particular clinical problems is limited by the frequency of presentation, although this is not a constraint in audits of special sessions, such as a diabetes clinic. The greatest constraints are the time it takes to observe and analyse the process of care, and the challenge of being observed by peers or experts. Paradoxically, this challenge is also one of the greatest strengths of this method.

On balance, the problems outweigh the advantages. Direct observation is used only infrequently in multicase audit because of the complexity and cost of analysis.

8 How to do it: data and methods II

THIS chapter outlines those audit methods that make use of several sources of data. The main audit methods in general practice, including those already described in the previous chapter, are summarized in Box 8.1. The use of practice data for routine performance monitoring, practice activity analysis, surveys and interviews and direct observation has already been considered. There remain three important approaches to audit that involve the collection of data from more than one source.

Box 8.1: Audit methods

- Routine performance monitoring
- Practice activity analysis
- Surveys and interviews
- Direct observation

- Confidential enquiries
- Use of tracers
- Practice visiting

Confidential enquiries

The confidential enquiry is a method relatively new to general practice. There are two separate but complementary approaches.

1 *Single significant events.* The examination of single significant events can be one of the most productive and effective forms of audit in general practice.[1] This approach developed from the 'random' case analysis used for teaching vocational registrars. The teaching method has been formalized and refined, mainly by ensuring that the scope for enquiry is broadened beyond the clinical notes used in case analysis to include the direct questioning of all concerned with a particular situation, and also by adopting a structured format for writing down the findings and conclusions.

   The examination of single significant events is concerned primarily with the reduction of clinical and organizational error, examples of which were described in Chapter 2. The aim of this method is to discover flaws in the process of care, the correction of which will have a beneficial effect on outcome for future patients.

   A case study involving all the members of one family and all the partners of a practice is described in detail in Case study 11. It may be helpful to read this case study at this point because it gives an indication of how such a situation can arise, how it can be investigated systematically by drawing on both the case notes and interviews with the people concerned, and what changes can result. Another very graphic example is given in the *Who killed Susan Thompson?* video and course book from the RCGP.[2]

2 *Aggregated significant events.* The examination of aggregated clinical and organizational significant events is usually external. The approach was pioneered by the Royal College of Obstetricians and Gynaecologists in the 1950s in their confidential enquiries into maternal and perinatal deaths,[3,4] and by the Royal College of Surgeons of England in the 1980s enquiring into perioperative deaths[5] (*see* Chapter 4). This approach is now being introduced into general practice. For example, DHAs routinely enquire into deaths from cervical cancer in women; an important part of these audits involves a detailed exploration of the screening process and of the events that may have led to a delay in the diagnosis in the setting of general practice. In future, aggregated data from significant incidents are likely to be collected and used by practices themselves. The choice of subject is important: the resources required to achieve a good result can be justified only if the error can be reduced significantly. Examples that fulfil this criterion include delay in the diagnosis of cases of meningitis, error in the treatment of an acute attack in asthmatic children, and the inappropriate management of acute chest pain.

Method

As the use of this method is wholly dependent on confidence and trust, it is essential that every member of a practice team who may become involved agrees to the audit *before* a single case is examined. Significant incidents and events are liable to reflect on care provided by certain individuals, and careless handling of audit can cause offence, damage confidence or result in non-cooperation.

The confidential enquiry is likely to become part of every practice team's performance monitoring procedures, and should be viewed as contributing to the practice's overall purpose or 'mission'. Seen in this context, the establishment of precise procedures suitable for any particular practice is a function of its practice management (*see* Chapter 10). However, the guidelines shown in Box 8.2 may help a practice team to determine what its approach should be.

It is essential to specify the purpose of confidential enquiries in writing, so that there is no possibility of misunderstanding. There are two basic purposes:

Box 8.2: Guidelines for practice confidential enquiries

- Specify the purpose.
- Establish confidentiality rules.
- Designate responsibility.
- Make arrangements for identifying significant events.
- Collect the evidence.
- Consider the results.
- Make necessary changes.

---

1 To seek to learn from the exercise and so secure improvement.
2 To apportion responsibility.

If the intention is to secure improvement – which is the only sensitive way of using the method – it must be made clear that the temptation in individual cases to apportion blame will not be allowed.

Establishing the ground rules for confidentiality is an equally important task. The general principles of confidentiality in audit should apply (as described in Chapter 11), but in addition the practice team may choose to retain the results of any confidential enquiry within the practice. Alternatively, a practice may choose to release anonymized data to the MAAG or others at its discretion. In some cases, the use of anonymized patient files should be considered within a practice, to protect either the patient or an individual health professional. This is probably more appropriate in larger practices, where some of the practice team may not have been involved in the case, than in smaller practices where it is likely that everyone will know of the initial problem.

It is helpful to have one named person take responsibility for organizing and conducting confidential enquiries. This person should collect data on all incidents, and decide which are to be explored further. The value of assigning responsibility is that the individual concerned will gain experience in the method. The named person should also be accountable to the partnership or practice team. The person responsible may wish to consult about individual cases, especially if a health professional in another discipline within the practice team was involved.

The method of choosing and collecting cases should be one that all members of the practice team know can operate. Incidents may be reported from a variety of sources, for example a patient complaint, a complaint by a partner or member of staff, by a local hospital or the social services, or through the practice's routine performance monitoring. The most important question to ask when choosing cases is: 'By looking at this event in more detail, is it likely that we will learn anything that will help avoid future error or otherwise secure improvement?'.

The key to a successful confidential enquiry lies in collecting the evidence. The relevant facts may be in the patient's records, documented in the appointment system or visiting books, or may be obtained by interviewing the individuals concerned. The presentation of the case history and the findings will form the basis for subsequent discussion.

Ideally the discussion should involve the whole practice team, so that everyone can learn. However, an incident involving technical clinical matters should be discussed by either the medical members of the practice or the medical and nursing staff together. It is essential that the individual who has carried out the enquiry should *not* chair the discussion, but should present the case, being prepared to clarify aspects of the history or findings as necessary.

It is important to record the conclusions, and particularly any proposals for change, because they may have wider implications for the practice. Such proposals should be fed back through the practice manager to the partnership for further consideration as part of the normal management process.

In the course of several confidential enquiries it may become clear that certain individuals have patterns of performance that are not satisfactory. If this should occur, it is important that the practice uses procedures separate from those of audit to manage the situation. The established machinery within the practice for investigating complaints about misconduct or persistently poor performance must be used. Members of a practice team have an ethical duty to ensure that patients are not put at unnecessary risk by the seriously deficient performance of an individual.

Use of tracers

In assessing the quality of care it is impossible to examine in detail every aspect of the work of individual clinicians or practice teams. The use of 'tracer' conditions may help to overcome this problem. A tracer is a single clinical condition, either a symptom or a disease entity, which is chosen to explore aspects of performance, usually by external review. In assessing the process and outcomes of care, the tracer condition chosen may be held to be representative of quality in similar conditions which are not being assessed. In Case study 7, hypertension was used as a tracer condition to demonstrate the standard of care of chronic illness in a practice.

To be effective, tracers should meet the criteria shown in Box. 8.3.

Box 8.3: 'Tracer' criteria

- The condition should be easy to define.
- The condition should be amenable to improvement by medical care.
- There should be a sound basis for discriminating between good and unsatisfactory care for the condition.

- The effects of non-medical factors on the condition should be adequately understood.
- The condition should yield enough patients for audit.

Source: Kessner et al., 1973[6]

As multipractice audits have become more common, tracers are used with increasing frequency. The use of tracers requires skill and resources for data handling, analysis and feedback, and therefore such audits are likely to be implemented by MAAGs and DHAs, which have the facilities to handle them.

Practice visiting

The third method of audit described in this chapter involves a visit made to a practice by local peers or external assessors. This approach was founded on the external assessment of teaching practices by visiting peers. It was initially developed by the RCGP, but is used today by the Joint Committee on Postgraduate Training for General Practice (JCPTGP) and regional postgraduate organizations for the selection of training practices. MAAGs and local audit groups are using methods equivalent to a practice visit as a means of helping to establish audit in general practices in their own areas.

Method

In some cases peer inspections can be relatively informal, but for most cases the method is more formalized. One of the best known is the RCGP's[7] *What Sort of Doctor?* method, in which four areas of practice are considered to be indicative of performance: professional values, accessibility, clinical competence and the ability to communicate. Data illustrating these aspects of performance can be obtained from routine statistics kept by the practice, clinical records, videos of consultations and interviews with the health professionals concerned. In New Zealand a patient's representative is included in the visiting team, and data are also sought from patients about satisfaction with care given.

A further description of the method is beyond the scope of this book, because practice visiting is an external audit. However, practitioners who are members of MAAGs and others who may be interested in the method will find that detailed information is available from the office of the regional director for postgraduate education in general practice, the JCPTGP (which carries out regular organizational audits of regional postgraduate organizations for accreditation purposes) and the RCGP,[8] which has detailed documentation on the data required of a practice in connection with the assessments made for fellowship of the College.

Summary

Audit method and data collection are interrelated. They are the heart of audit. In this and the preceding chapter we have attempted to show the range of data already available in the average practice, and how simple methods of data collection can make more data available relatively easily. The most popular audit methods, especially practice activity analysis and the analysis of individual cases, are within the scope of any practice team and, taken together, they make a useful starting point.

9 How to do it: analysing and
feeding back information

The data collection grid

WHATEVER the initial objectives and the methods chosen, any audit will produce a considerable amount of data. Example 9.1 gives a hypothetical situation.

Example 9.1

An audit was carried out in one practice of people aged over 75 years who were taking antihypertensive therapy. The practice team identified 40 cases, from the practice computer, the repeat prescription system, or through the opportunistic recording of cases when seen by the doctor. The basic demographic data about the patients were recorded: age, sex and so on. Recording the time and level of the last blood pressure reading was important, as was recording the types of treatment and iatrogenic problems. These data were collected by practice activity analysis and a series of interviews. Each of the 40 cases yielded 20 items of data, which were set out on a data selection grid (*see* Fig. 9.1).

As a result there were 800 (40 × 20) boxes or cells to complete in the grid. Not all the items in these boxes required 'Yes' or 'No' answers: some included a range of options, such as marital status (single, widowed or married (S, W or M)) or the type of drug therapy, labelled a, b or c, thereby substantially increasing the potential number of data items.

Example 9.1 illustrates several points.

1 A considerable quantity of data can be generated by audit even when only a small number of cases are being examined. This underlines the importance of starting small and planning the audit according to the skills and data-handling resources available. It also reinforces the point made in Chapter 7 that a data item should be collected only if it is necessary.

2 Any attempt at analysis will be frustrated unless a suitable method of organizing the data has been devised at the planning stage. In general, and particularly for smaller audits, all the data should be entered into a grid drawn on paper (*see* Fig. 9.1). This gives an overview essential to understanding the nature and quality of the information that can be derived from the data. In practices where there is appropriate computer

	1	2	3	4	5	6	→ 20
	Age	Sex	Drug	Marital status	BP recorded		
Case 1	94	M	A	S	Y		
Case 2	90	M	B	W	Y		
Case 3	87	F	C	M	N		
↓ 40							

Figure 9.1   Data collection grid

software and expertise, computerized spreadsheets can be used; for larger data sets a simple analysis package is essential.

3 The data collected should be 'clean'. Inconsistencies need to be identified, for example:

- cases in which the age lies outside the chosen age range
- misrecordings of sex or marital status
- unusual combinations of events due either to error or to an unusual care pattern.

The analysis

The analysis must reflect the aims of the audit. If the purpose was to examine the drugs that seemed to cause side-effects in older people on anti-hypertensive therapy, this should be the priority of the analysis. One of the dangers of computerized analysis is the capacity to examine many items. The laws of probability ensure that the more data that are examined, the greater the likelihood will be of revealing interesting patterns. However, this will distract from the original aim of the audit, and analysis should always be focused.

The first step in any analysis is to examine the frequency of occurrence of each item or event. Thus, using Example 9.1, eight out of the 40 people may be widowed, and 15 out of 40 may be taking two or more drugs. Each of these numbers could be expressed as percentages, although percentages should not be used unless there are 50 or more cases in any data set.

The next step is to construct a table that shows the range of each item of

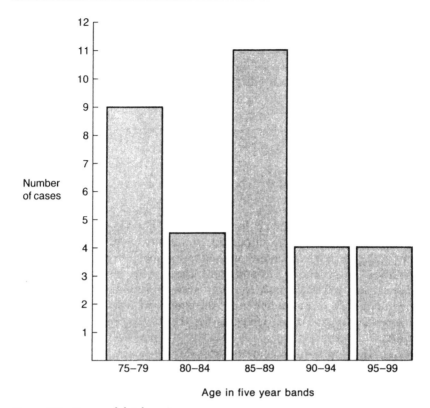

Figure 9.2   Range of database items

data collected (Fig. 9.2). The point of this exercise is to highlight unusual occurrences; analysis can then be focused on these events.

If some of the key data items or variables are not well represented within a range (for instance, there may be only one person in each annual age group) grouping the cases together in a logical way that fits an agreed convention can overcome this problem. Ages can be grouped in five-year bands: 75–79, 80–84, 85–89 and so on.

As a result, part of the analysis should be to produce one or more tables containing only the data required. For instance, the data in Fig. 9.1 can be summarized as shown in Fig. 9.3.

Statistical analysis

Summary statistics based on simple techniques, such as proportions or means, together with frequencies or counts, form the basis for much of the

Age (years)	Married	Single	Total	BP recorded	Antihypertensive prescribed
75–79	9	3	12	13	0
80–84	4	2	6	10	1
85–89	3	7	10	2	1
90–94	2	6	8	1	0
95–99	1	3	4	2	
Total	19	21	40	28	2

Figure 9.3   Data presentation card

analysis required for clinical audit. Complex statistical analysis is unnecessary for the majority of single-practice audits. The idea of undertaking a statistical analysis may be offputting to certain team members. Consequently, this section has concentrated on simple methods of analysis and the techniques of generating information; those who have an interest in statistical analysis may wish to apply such techniques to results where appropriate. The short reading list at the end of the book contains some of the more useful statistical references for those who wish to explore this option.

Recent developments in computer software packages offer an alternative approach to manual statistical analysis. It is useful to have access to an analysis package that will facilitate comparisons. For instance, when examining iatrogenic problems in frail, elderly people receiving antihypertensive therapy, as in Example 9.1, it may be necessary to detect any differences between men and women at different ages. Two groups of patients, male and female, would have to be selected and then tables constructed such as those shown in Fig. 9.4.

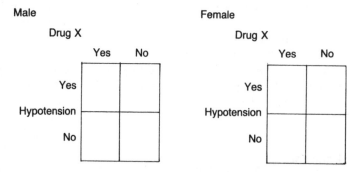

Figure 9.4   The tabulation that would show the distribution of hypotensive symptoms in males and females, receiving or not receiving drug X

Comparisons could also be made with patients who are *not* taking the drug in question, i.e. untreated controls. However, the volume of work involved if such comparisons have to be done manually (aided by a calculator) is large. Fortunately, the software now available can be run on a microcomputer; one such package is called EpiInfo, the details of which are included in the references to this chapter at the end of the book.[1] Alternatively, the MAAG or local audit group should be able to provide this level of support.

Presentation of data

The analysis of data produces results that need to be converted into information the practice team can understand and to which they can relate. Many health professionals are not used to interpreting data and are discouraged by tables that summarize many facts. Trends or insights should be presented in a visual way that communicates the information effectively.

To return to Example 9.1: suppose there are six different permutations of therapeutic regimen that the patients under study could be taking:

Thiazides only	4
Methyldopa	2
Beta-blockers	10
ACE inhibitors	4
Beta-blockers and thiazide	12
None	8

This information can be presented graphically by the use of a pie chart, as in Fig. 9.5, or as a bar chart, as in Fig. 9.6. Simple graphics programs can be run on personal computers: EpiInfo is easy to use in this respect. Alternatively, local schools or colleges are often willing to provide graphical skills.

There are sound reasons for spending time on ensuring the acceptability of the data presentation.

1 The information may be disturbing to some team members. No practice can provide consistently high quality in all aspects of health care. The purpose of audit is to highlight particular aspects of performance, and inevitably there will be times when elements of performance will fall below stated objectives. Whatever the mechanism the practice team has for feeding back audit results, it needs to take into account the potential for finding uncomfortable results and how those results are to be handled. The management framework necessary to ensure that such

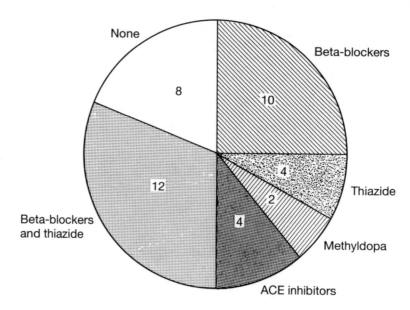

Figure 9.5   Data displayed as pie chart

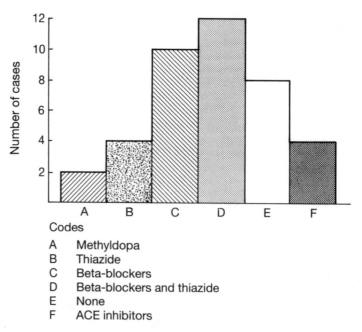

Figure 9.6   Data displayed as bar chart

presentations lead to effective and planned changes is discussed in Chapter 10. Case study 10 provides an illustration of what happens when such a framework does not exist.

2 Effective presentation assists accurate interpretation (*see* Chapter 7); in Case study 15, an audit of the care of patients with diabetes shows how presentation can help a practice to distinguish between an improvement in patient care resulting from better drug management and an improvement in the standard of record-keeping. If it had been presented in the form of tables, it might have been harder for colleagues to interpret the information correctly.

Summary

The purpose of feedback is to allow health professionals to compare the information obtained with their initial explicit standards, to debate the issues raised, to question performance and to make proposals for improvement where appropriate. Without effective practice management to ensure that such proposals are implemented and that changes are monitored (to confirm that improvement is attained and maintained), the process of audit is pointless. For this reason, in Chapter 10 the management context for the practice team and for the audit is discussed, and the importance of setting audit in a wider context is emphasized.

10 Management – achieving the change: changing habits

THIS book began by emphasizing that clinical audit cannot and should not be regarded as anything other than an integral part of modern general practice. Internal audit provides the means by which a practice can regularly and systematically monitor its own progress against standards which it itself has chosen. The whole point of external audit is to help a practice see where it stands in relation to others and, where appropriate, to use the results to bring about improvements.

Previous chapters have shown that the basic methods of audit are straightforward. As was established in Chapter 2, the tricky areas are in the before and after, that is, in motivating people to use audit purposefully in the first place, and to use the results of audit constructively when they show that change is necessary. Motivating, monitoring performance and achieving change are all functions of modern practice management.

So why is there a problem? The answer lies partly in the perception of clinical audit as an add-on activity, an optional extra to mainline practice, but mainly in the state of development of practice management itself.

Practice management is still widely perceived as being concerned with simple administrative and organizational activities and tasks only indirectly concerned with clinical care. Audit, and all it stands for, does not figure in this view of practice management. However, things are slowly changing. There is a growing number of practices which see in practice management a way of making patient care more effective and life in general practice more satisfying. This explains why there has been growth in the sophistication of management skills within general practice in doctors, nurses, and particularly in practice managers. This in turn has made it possible for general practice to accommodate, for instance, fundholding, commissioning and the pursuit of clinically effective practice in ways that ten years ago would not have seemed possible.

General practice today is in the midst of a major cultural change. Part of this change includes general practitioners accepting the close and distinct relationship between clinical management and the management of people and organizations. Many find this difficult, which is why a whole chapter is devoted to it.

Management functions

The starting point is to recall the basic management functions. These are set out in Box 10.1.

Box 10.1: Basic management functions

- Recognize the inevitability of change.
- Help the organization deal with uncertainty while moving towards overall goals.
- Introduce stability and clarify direction in situations of rapid change or conflict.
- Underpin the professional activity.
- Ensure that the clinical process is supported by groups of appropriate and effectively functioning staff.
- Apply rules appropriately and consistently.

Source: Irvine and Irvine (1996)[1]

In general practice there remains some confusion about the role of doctors as managers, not least because of the many other roles they occupy. General practitioners are the owners of their businesses and most commonly hold the legal and financial responsibility, both for the practice as an organization and for its role in the community – the delivery of effective health care to the registered population. General practitioners still take the key decisions, both on the direction the practice should develop and on the policy framework for allocating resources. At the same time they are the principal providers of the key direct services to patients. Both these roles and the basic management functions set out in Box 10.1 demand a high level of management skills and attributes. These are set out in Box 10.2.

Box 10.2: Management skills and attributes

- *Human skills*, such as being a group leader, building and maintaining a team and selecting staff.
- *Technical skills*: decision-making, priority setting, budgeting and planning, forecasting, establishing communications and information systems.
- *Political skills*, such as understanding and using authority, wielding personal power and personal influence to advantage, creating the conditions for change, identifying organizational opportunities.
- *Skills concerned with an ability to take an overview and see the enterprise as a whole.*

Source: Irvine and Irvine (1996)[1]

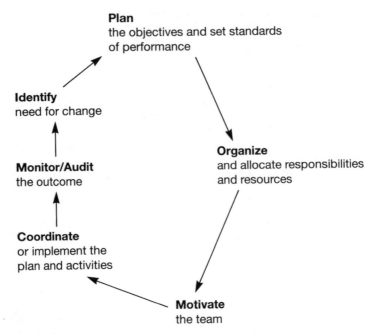

Figure 10.1   The management cycle

Clearly, these skills and attributes require general practitioners to be aware of the key levers in the management process for turning the results of audit into effective change. These levers are planning, teamwork (encompassing leadership, delegation and motivation) and managing change, and are often shown in cyclical form (Fig. 10.1) – the so-called management cycle.

Planning

Planning is the starting point of the management cycle, as it is of the audit process. Planning is necessary because it gives a sense of direction, focuses the resources of the practice on key objectives, and provides answers to the following questions:

- Where are we now?
- Where do we want to be?
- How can we get there?
- How will we know when we have arrived?
- If we do not arrive, will we know why?

This process of reviewing a practice and making its purposes explicit is fundamental; it is also important to share agendas. If the career expectations of individual members of the practice team differ, and these differences are not explained or monitored, conflict may result. Lack of agreement about the aims of a practice can cause resistance to change. In Case study 14 audit was used to revive a demoralized and frustrated practice team; it provides an example of how the integration of audit results and management processes is essential to practice direction.

Today, general practitioners are subject to a changing culture in which it is likely that professional and financial rewards will be given to those who are considered to be effective providers of primary care. Effective care is invariably planned care. Planned care is proactive and explicit; unplanned care is reactive, leaving much unstated, such that other professionals would find it difficult to understand either the process of care in a practice and/or its objectives.

The choice between planned and unplanned care may have practical consequences. For example, obtaining substantial financial backing from financial institutions may be difficult without evidence of coherent planning, especially in written form. Similarly, seeking support from health authorities for expanding services (or the maintenance of existing services) is unlikely to be successful without a clear indication of what is to be achieved and how.

Benefits of development planning

It is now common for the planning stage of a management cycle to be written down. A 'development plan' or 'business plan' is the description of a practice's existing situation, the team's aspirations, and the means of getting from here to there and assessing whether it has arrived.[2,3] Illustrative headings and a structure for a conventional development plan are shown in Fig. 10.2. Making the plan explicit clarifies the issues facing a practice team and enables it to identify workable solutions. The thought and discussion involved in generating a business plan are as important as the outcome. Writing down a development plan is a visible sign of a planning process. It can provide a secure framework within which the practice's audit activities can be planned and prioritized.

However, the benefits of a business plan need to be tangible to ensure commitment. Such benefits are listed in Box 10.3.

Box 10.3: The benefits of development planning

A development plan:

- ensures that the actions of the practice are fitted to its strategic direction

- can help build a feeling of corporateness, without discouraging personal innovation
- identifies explicitly the choices and the changes that have to be made
- focuses on balancing the aspirations of the practice, in terms of the services it wishes to provide, against the resources available, in terms of money, staff, estate and equipment
- identifies which factors are critical to success
- requires the practice to assess explicitly the risk factors involved in its plans
- identifies the different consumers of the practice's services (including the staff) and allows more effective and targeted marketing.

1 Overall purpose 'Mission' and aims	Where are we now and where are we going, broadly and more specificallly?
Activities	What do we have to do to get there?
2 Resources Time Data Money Organizations People Systems Capital stock Protocols	What do we need to get there?
3 Constraints/Strengths *Identify constraints* Internal and external to the practice	What are the current constraints and what are we likely to meet in the future?
Identify strengths Internal and external to the practice	What factors are working in our favour now and what factors are likely to arise in the future?
4 Monitoring of performance The standard setting/performance review cycle	How will we know when and if we have got there? If we don't make it, will we know why?

Source: Irvine D (1990)[4]

Figure 10.2   The development plan

How to plan

In devising and drafting a development plan all team members should be involved, particularly those party to the management of the practice. It is essential that a practice devotes 'protected' time to this process. Time is necessary for effective brainstorming: ideas should not be constrained by resource considerations or political necessity.

Different groupings of team members can generate different perspectives of practice aims: for example, nurses, receptionists or partners can meet separately to brainstorm. When each group has finalized its ideas, all groups should meet to discuss them. An external facilitator can often help team members to overcome the traditional relationships and modes of expression within a practice. Although the process can be time-consuming, a general practice team with a common purpose or 'mission' is strong.

As the development plan will be the result of team effort, the process requires delegation to specific groups and individuals.

Teamwork

The implementation of teamwork among doctors generally and general practitioners in particular remains patchy.[3,5] There are important reasons for this:

- General practitioners, by the nature of their training and their jobs, acquire attitudes and a professional ethos that favours independent action, often at the expense of concerted effort. This ethos stresses the value of personal rather than shared care.
- Common, explicit team objectives, criteria and standards are frequently missing, usually because the value of an active planning process in primary care, which includes performance review and audit, is still not widely recognized.
- Multidisciplinary audit, and the joint monitoring of patients whose care is shared by all team members, is still very underdeveloped.

It is clear that mutual support for and understanding of personal and team goals, and a climate of trust in which honest communication is encouraged, are vital to effective audit. This is particularly true when presenting potentially uncomfortable findings, as Chapter 9 emphasized. Effective teams include members who are encouraged to develop skills, apply what they learn and contribute to the success of the practice by using their individual talents and knowledge to achieve a common purpose.

Irvine D (1997)[6] has suggested that doctors are most likely to achieve their plans and maintain clinical excellence when they practice in teams which:

- are able to show leadership
- have clear values and standards
- are collectively committed to quality
- foster learning
- care for each other.

He states that effective clinical teams are committed to:

- continuing quality assurance
- personal and professional team development
- a focus on educational activity
- good internal management
- a 'no blame' culture
- an ability to test themselves against others.

This requires leadership, delegation and motivational skills.

Leadership

The capacity to show leadership is crucial in management. It is very difficult to be an effective manager without being a good leader, although it is less true that you cannot be a good leader without being a good manager. Handy (1994)[7] defines a leader as someone who shapes and shares a vision which gives point to the work of others.

Because of a cultural distaste for direct leadership, few general practitioners handle policy and strategic management comfortably. Indeed, in order to disguise the leadership demands of management, practices often have a very broad structure in which the areas of personal responsibility and accountability may be left deliberately vague. Partnership agreements nowadays are built on the basis of equality and certainly do not carry within them any means of sanctioning aberrant behaviour beyond serious professional misconduct. As a consequence, wide variations in the standard of clinical performance are tolerated.

However, even within this flat approach it is possible to allocate responsibility to partners and to identify consensus policies. Clinical standards and operational policies can be developed, indicators for hospital referrals can be redefined, and levels of expenditure and methods of charging can be written. In partnerships today there is frequently a reluctance to take the lead because of fear of being seen as putting oneself above one's peers. There is also anxiety about the amount of time, effort and energy that may be involved. However, if these are overriding considerations, then perhaps the practice should look to others outside the partnership team who have the time, energy and commitment to create the leadership function that is so vital, particularly in the application of change arising from audit.

Delegation

One of the most important aspects of leadership is the capacity to delegate effectively and appropriately. Delegation is an arrangement whereby certain team members take on particular tasks or roles. Delegation can reveal a hidden core of resources and can be used to put existing skills to better effect. The appropriate delegation of administrative tasks can release other team members to perform the strategic tasks for which they have the expertise and for which they are able to take responsibility.

Delegation can increase personal development, which results in greater job satisfaction and the enhancement of one's skills. A receptionist given total responsibility for complete tasks, such as dealing with all aspects of new patient registrations, may perform them more effectively than when handling a whole series of disparate activities. Delegation confers ownership; ownership often leads to innovation and pride in a job well done.

There is no easy way to learn to delegate. In general, it is important to ensure that the task being delegated is clearly defined, and that appropriate support and authority are given. It is also important to ensure that the delegator understands the needs to let go, to accept mistakes as learning opportunities for all, and to praise success. Most importantly, supervision and monitoring appropriate to the task should be given. Both delegator and delegatee need to feel confident about the tasks being delegated. The rules of good delegation are set out in Box 10.4.

Box 10.4: The rules of good delegation

1 Try not to do the work others can do.
2 Always make clear the purpose of the delegation.
3 Agree the arrangements for control and monitoring with the delegatee beforehand.
4 Delegate the whole job wherever possible.
5 Make sure there are adequate resources to carry out the tasks.
6 Use language to delegate that is clear and free from technical jargon and check that the delegatee understands the task.
7 If mistakes arise, criticize constructively and in private.
8 Ask others if they know of areas that could be delegated.
9 Be aware that although the delegatee can be made accountable to the delegator for the delegated task, the delegator cannot give up final responsibility.
10 Take advantage of any criticism that may come from delegation.

Source: Irvine (1995)[9]

Motivation

In order to ensure appropriate teamwork and effective delegation the leader's and manager's function is to motivate others. An awareness of what motivates people and how to encourage them to work to their optimum is vital. Normal mature adults seek stimulation in their work and are anxious to use and develop their capabilities. If they work for years in organizations that tightly prescribe their work activities, allowing little initiative and discretion, this capacity atrophies. They take refuge in the routine or seek stimulation in social relationships on the job, in the hours, in the holidays or in the contact with patients.

Hertzberg (1996)[8] has written extensively on the difference between hygiene factors and the motivating factors. Hygiene factors are those needs that can be seen as stemming from a human being's animal nature, the built-in drive to avoid pain from the environment, including drives such as hunger. The motivating factors are those that relate to the need to achieve, and through achievement to experience psychological growth. Box 10.5 summarizes these two sets of factors.

Box 10.5: Hygiene and motivating factors

Hygiene factors
- Company policy
- Administration
- Supervision
- Interpersonal relationships
- Working conditions
- Salary, status and security

Motivating factors
- Achievement
- Recognition for achievement
- The work itself
- Responsibility, growth or advancement

Concentrating on hygiene factors is insufficient to produce job satisfaction. Good conditions of service, good pay and efficient processes alone will not result in a contented and motivated workforce, if there is not job satisfaction and responsibility. Thus it is clear that the psychology of motivation is very complicated, and the psychological contract that each person has with their job varies. However, improving the design of somebody's job, rotating them from one task to another, enlarging their job and giving them autonomy all contribute to motivation. Feedback is also important. Staff need to know how they are doing and they need to be shown appreciation.

Above all, good motivation, like good teamworking, requires consistency of management. Consistency in management – or rather the lack of it – is possibly one of the biggest problems in general practice. Differences between partners can create confusion and frustration among employees, and make them feel that the efficiency and effectiveness of the whole practice is reduced. It can create a need to spend additional energy and time, and therefore money, to meet the individual doctor's idiosyncrasies.

General practice is developing fast as a work organization as well as a profession. The general practice of the 1990s and beyond will require a competent, confident staff who are offered opportunities to grow in their work and to develop new knowledge and skills. To manage change appropriately such a motivated workforce is vital. The mushroom theory of management – 'leave them in the dark and drop manure on them' – will no longer do. Good managers help subordinates feel strong and responsible, reward them well and properly for good performance, and foster a good strong sense of teamwork, which is what motivation is all about.

Managing change

After establishing an ethos of forward planning, and developing teamworking, the third major element *en route* to the effective translation of the results of audit into changed behaviour is the management of change. Much has been written on this topic.[10,11] This is not an end in itself, but only one component of a broader process. As already said, good managers are rarely taken by surprise. They plan ahead, they scan the horizon, they look for all possible pitfalls and decide upon alternative strategies and tactics. If change is required good managers are able to handle it, having motivated their staff and delegated appropriately. They will have a strong team to help them. Crisis management, which is the only alternative to good change management, leads to short-term solutions which can be extremely draining on the personnel involved, particularly in general practice, where team members are already subject to considerable stress.

Managing change is more difficult now as organizations become less hierarchical, more fluid and more technology based, with less clear-cut demarcation lines and much more complex decision-making processes. General practice has a particular problem: as a structure it has retained its traditional pattern of work and relationships almost unscathed. Only now is it beginning to feel the force of changed societal values and attitudes towards how organizations work and how skills are valued. Some practices continue to work on traditional bureaucratic principles, relying on the old reverence for doctors and loyalty that is given rather than earned, work being seen as a privilege rather than a mere occupation. Some of these values are worth trying to retain, but most of them will go because the world has changed. But in moving from the old, the new must be based on firm foundations. This is not always easy.

There are certain clear stages in managing change and they are usually set out as in Box 10.6.

Box 10.6: Stages in managing change

1 Understanding the change.
2 Organizing the implementation.
3 Evaluating the change.

It is essential at an early stage to communicate the need for change and to assess its impact on those likely to be involved. If it is a change resulting from audit, appropriate planning will have ensured that the team members likely to be affected will have been involved in collecting the data and interpreting the results (*see* Chapter 4). This can help engage commitment to the proposed change, as can ensuring appropriate rewards.

People respond to change in two ways, as either innovators or adopters. Innovators are those who are not frightened by new ideas. They also tend not to recognize any of the fears that those with whom they are communicating may experience. Adopters are the recipients of other people's bright ideas, and frequently tend to be left behind in understanding where the proposed changes have come from and where they are heading. They tend to become anxious and therefore resistant to change. Either way, it helps to present innovation or change as a benefit for patients. In developing changes resulting from audit it is important, therefore, that the adopters are not left out.

Moreover, the costs of change can be enormous and are frequently played down. They must be weighed in the balance before the changes are decided upon, and at the same time they need to be identified before the change is implemented so that strategies can be devised to deal with them.

Development and training is of major importance in ensuring effective change management. It has this importance because of the role it plays in helping people understand what Glouberman and Mintzberg[12] call 'the other actors in the system'. Ensuring effective delegation and reducing the amount of error is itself a major reason for investing appropriately in development and training. It is also a sign of respect for the individual and an intrinsic part of the motivational factors that make people feel self-disciplined and committed, but all too often this sort of investment goes by the board.

Summary

As this chapter shows, the management of general practice requires the same techniques and skills as the management of any business. These involve being able to make the right choice between competing demands and deciding upon the most appropriate use of resources. Good practice management includes knowing how to delegate and how to communicate effectively; how to plan and set objectives and how to monitor achievement. It includes knowing how to lead and how to support; how to encourage and motivate; how to cooperate and how to take responsibility; how to take decisions and how to exercise authority.

The effective management of a practice is vital to improve the standards of patient care and to ensure that those standards have been achieved. Without effective audit this is not possible, and without the management framework within which audit can function and its results be implemented, audit is worthless.

11 Confidentiality

No guidance on audit would be complete without considering confidentiality with respect to both patients and health professionals.

Confidentiality and the patient

In any practice audit should be conducted within the framework of confidentiality that already regulates clinical care. General Medical Council (GMC) guidelines[1] state that confidentiality should be preserved, except when the release of information may be specifically permitted, provided that the doctors can justify their action. There are similar guidelines from the United Kingdom Council for Nursing, Midwifery and Health Visiting (UKCC)[2] governing the relationship of nurses with their patients. Clinical confidentiality may extend beyond the individual doctor to other practitioners and members of the practice team concerned with the care of a patient. In general, it is accepted by the GMC and by lay organizations, both in this country and abroad, that it is in the best interests of patients that health professionals within a practice should have access to medical records in confidence for the purpose of improving standards of patient care, i.e. for *internal* audit.

However, audit is not always internal: it may involve access to patient records by visiting peers, as in visits to training practices. The GMC has given guidance on training practice visiting that is relevant and can be applied to all practice audit activity. In its annual report in 1986,[3] the GMC recommended that the existing arrangements for training practice inspections should continue, but specified that all doctors carrying out such inspections should act with sensitivity and discretion, and be conscious that they are bound by professional secrecy. The GMC also recommended that each training practice should ensure that all of its patients were informed of the circumstances in which their medical records might be disclosed to other doctors, for educational purposes. Such information can be given to patients via practice leaflets and notices in the surgeries. The GMC concluded with a statement that all patients have the right to refuse access to their medical records for audit purposes.

Confidentiality and doctors

During the operation of clinical audit doctors will be concerned that their names are protected. This concern is acknowledged in the DoH health circulars on audit.[4,5] This aspect of audit and confidentiality can be considered at two levels: within the practice, and in the relationship between the practice and the outside world.

It is important that a practice establishes policy guidance on confidentiality and internal audit because internal audit could reveal aspects of individual performance that previously had not been obvious or thought important. There are two ways of managing this situation.

1 The practice can decide that all matters revealed by an internal audit should usually remain private, especially if the performance of individual health professionals is concerned. The uncovering of seriously deficient performance must, however, be an exception (*see* below). The practice should also decide what to publish, and what form publication should take.

2 The practice should consider an internal policy on anonymization. This is likely to apply to the confidential enquiry audit (*see* Chapter 8) in which a particular health professional's name may not be relevant to the purpose and conduct of the audit. The easiest way to handle this aspect in practice is to apply the 'need to know' principle on each individual occasion.

In terms of the relationship between the practice and the outside world, it is important to determine MAAG policies on confidentiality and to ensure that the practice policy complies. In general, MAAGs and any other external auditing bodies are advised to use anonymized data wherever possible. GMSC and RCGP policy is that nothing should be sent from a practice to an MAAG which would identify either the general practitioner or the patient. Legal advice has confirmed that information held by MAAGs could be subpoenaed by the courts.

It cannot be emphasized too strongly that, particularly at the level of the practice, privacy is of the utmost importance if honesty and trust are to be combined in the pursuit of improvement.

Confidentiality and professional obligation

One of the most common questions asked about the operation of audit is: 'What should happen if less than satisfactory performance is revealed?'. This sharpens even more the question of privacy and anonymity. The GMC has recently issued guidance to doctors to cover the situation when a practitioner has to comment on a colleague's professional practice. Although this situation can arise in a number of circumstances, it is likely to be of particular relevance in audit procedures. It is worthwhile noting in full the GMC's guidance to doctors[1] in such circumstances:

'You must protect patients when you believe that a colleague's conduct, performance or health is a threat to them.

Before taking action, you should do your best to find out the facts. Then, if necessary, you must tell someone from an employing authority or from a regulatory body. Your comments about colleagues must be honest. If you are not sure what to do, ask an experienced colleague. The safety of patients must come first at all times.'

This is the guidance that all practices should follow.

12 Audit – looking ahead

AUDIT in general practice has come a long way in the five years since the first edition of this book was published. This is a remarkable achievement for both practices and the MAAGs, given that, unlike hospital specialists, there is no contractual obligation on general practitioners to take part in audit.

The way forward was set out recently in the report of the Primary Health Care Clinical Audit Working Group of the DoH's Clinical Outcomes Group.[1] This concluded that:

- achieving and maintaining good quality primary health care will most likely happen where practices are themselves committed to the philosophy, principles and methods of quality improvement and assurance
- clinical audit should be seen as one of the key instruments for assessing and ensuring quality
- clinical audit should continue to be professionally led. It should 'follow the patient'. Sometimes, therefore, clinical audit will be multidisciplinary, sometimes unidisciplinary, and sometimes multisectoral, as when, for example, hospital care is also involved
- the means must be found to bring patients' perspectives to bear on audit whenever possible
- the effectiveness of clinical audit in general practice is critically bound up with the quality of teamworking and practice management. Practitioners who know how to work together and manage themselves well will make best use of clinical audit
- new and improved computer record systems in general practice will make the collection and analysis of data even easier in future
- practices, as well as building internal audit into their everyday work, must be prepared to have the quality of their care assessed and compared against others through external audit and review.

We agree with these conclusions. We would add simply that in our experience most practices in the United Kingdom today want to do the best they can for their patients, and such practices are most enthusiastic about the use of audit. For them, clinical audit is essential to their central purpose, both now and for the future.

Section II

13 Introduction to Case Studies

THE second half of this book is devoted to descriptions of audits that were collected by the contributors from their own and neighbouring practices for the first edition, and which are now updated and amended for the second edition. In one case the Case study is completely new. The case studies remain previously unpublished and are not the result of research work. They are varied in their complexity, rigour and success. They have been presented in a common format for ease of reference, but their strength lies in the reality of the situations they describe.

They provide a series of illustrations of the points made in Section I. They can be used as models or inspirations. They illustrate one or more of the benefits detailed in Chapter 2. The audits described use a variety of the data sources and methods described in Chapters 7 and 8.

Readers can read the case studies without reference to the text, or may prefer to refer to them as encountered as cross-references in Section I. For instance, Case study 11 is an example of a critical incident audit and it may be helpful to read it together with the section on critical incident enquiries in Chapter 8; when reading Case study 10, which illustrates practice activity analysis, it may be useful to read the section in Chapter 7 to expand upon the contents of the case study. References to relevant texts are given as appropriate, although the editors have resisted introducing too many in the interests of readability.

14   Case Studies

No.	Subject	Method
1	Reviewing the effectiveness of a 'well man' clinic and the consequent use of resources.	Practice activity using informal contact data
2	Reviewing the effectiveness of a screening programme for a practice's 'over 75s'.	Proforma
3	Reviewing the impact of a screening service with a practice standard for epilepsy care.	Self-administered patient questionnaire
4	Reducing clinical error by comparing performance with a practice standard for epilepsy care.	Records review
5	Improving the effectiveness of rubella immunization among adolescent girls.	Practice activity analysis
6	Reducing clinical error in the use of H_2-antagonists.	Case review
7	Demonstrating the standard of care in hypertension.	Tracer condition
8	Reviewing organizational error.	Organization review
9	An audit of high-risk hypertensives.	Computer review of patient lists
10	Identifying reasons for frustration and irritation.	1 Practice activity analysis 2 Patient satisfaction 3 Confidential enquiry
11	Reducing clinical and organizational error.	Confidential enquiry
12	Assessing effectiveness of a changed approach to the delivery of diabetes care.	Records review

13	Assessing patterns of referral practice.	Practice activity analysis using data collection sheet
14	Improving effectiveness and efficiency of rubella immunization.	Audit of process/ intermediate outcome using routine practice data
15	Improving glycaemic control in diabetic patients.	Disease index and patient records

Case Study 1

Subject of audit

A process audit reviewing the efficiency and effectiveness of a 'well man' clinic and the consequent use of resources, using practice activity analysis and routine practice data.

Background

A nurse-led 'well man' clinic had been established in the practice to offer health checks to men aged 30–60 years as part of the health promotion programme. The practice nurse had been given a major role in its planning and institution, protocol development and in implementation. A postal call and recall system was used to contact the selected population of men aged 30–60 years. A standard letter was produced which provided an appointment time, the aims of the clinic and a brief description of what would happen. Appointments were booked such that the clinic was in operation for one day of each week. A three-year cycle was planned for these health checks.

The administrative tasks were the responsibility of one of the reception staff. They included the identification of patients from the age–sex register, making appointments, sending out letters and recording the attenders and non-attenders.

Reason for the audit

As one of the partners remarked, 'It would be nice to say that this audit was part of a general policy of looking at what we were doing. Regrettably, most of us only look at our work when a problem is identified, and this audit was no different!'.

The doctors and nurses felt that the turnout at the clinic was low, particularly for younger men. Too much nurse time seemed to be lost in waiting for patients who were booked but did not turn up. The nurse also wondered if she was providing a valuable service – did she really pick up any significant illnesses or concerns among attenders?

Aims of audit

The audit was performed to test the impression that, in terms of turnout and positive findings by age, the clinic could be made more effective.

Methods

Routine practice activity data, entered into the appointment book and on to a specially designed proforma kept within the clinical record, were abstracted and analysed. In addition, when non-attenders at the clinics came to the surgery for another reason, they were asked why they had not attended the clinic, and their answers were collated.

Who carried out the audit?

One option was for a partner to conduct this audit. However, the task was given to the practice manager to delegate appropriately. The counting and initial analysis was carried out by the receptionist who had special responsibility for the clinic, and the further analysis by the practice manager, practice nurse and partners.

Results

The audit confirmed that turnout was very poor in the younger age group, but improved with the increasing age of patients (Table CS1.1).

Informal questioning by both doctors and nurses during other contact revealed the reasons for non-attendance. The clinic was held during working hours and, as most men saw no need for a health check because they felt well, they did not attend. However, many became interested when it was discussed with them, and arranged an appointment.

Table CS1.1   Turnout by age

Age (years)	Attenders (%)
30–39	37
40–49	45
50–59	55

Table CS1.2 Examples of frequency of positive findings by age (percentage of age group)

Findings	Age (years)		
	30–39	40–49	50–59
Urine abnormal	1.5	3	6
PEF abnormal	22	6	34
Blood pressure borderline (single reading)	22	7	32
Blood pressure raised	0	0	6
Non-smokers	62	43	33
Non-drinkers	6	9	22
Normal BMI	70	94	98
Smokers, at least 15 cigarettes/day	19	18	28
Drinkers, at least 30 units/week	20	17	12

The positive findings were difficult to interpret (Table CS1.2). 'Hard' factors, such as urine screening, had a minimal positive pick-up: less than 5% overall showed any abnormality. Several men were found to have borderline hypertension which required further checking. The majority of the men who had had their serum cholesterol measured were found to have a level above the norm, consequent with national research findings. 'Soft' data, relating to smoking, alcohol and body mass index, were obtained which formed the basis for further health education.

The analysis showed that the timing of the clinic was inconvenient, its purpose was not understood and it was not well advertised. The findings also demonstrated that further health education would be valuable in men with risk factors, such as cigarette smoking and excessive alcohol consumption.

Changes resulting from audit

It was obvious that major organizational changes were required.

1 The routine call and recall system was abandoned.
2 The clinic was advertised in the surgery.
3 Women attending for cervical cytology were informed of the service available for their partners.
4 Appointments were offered opportunistically when men attended for routine consultations. Thus, the overall allocation of appointments to a specific day was changed to a more flexible arrangement guided by the convenience of the patient and nurse.

The problem of getting young men interested in health education formed the basis of a practice educational meeting; the practice nurse has undertaken further educational courses in smoking cessation; and specific protocols, such as those for obesity management, have been developed.

Was the audit repeated?

It was important to see whether these developments produced any changes. The audit was repeated and revealed a far greater turnout of patients for these checks: over 90% of those who made appointments kept them. Consequently, the nurse was able to use her time more efficiently. Although the pick-up of positive findings revealed much the same outcomes, the nurse's confidence in dealing with men with risk factors (smoking, drinking and obesity) had increased. Subsequent audits should reveal whether changes in patient behaviour lead to fewer smokers, reduced alcohol consumption etc.

Comment

This audit is an example of a simple practice activity analysis (*see* Chapter 7) and helps to answer the question of efficiency. It is ideal for monitoring the activity produced by a 'well man' clinic.

This audit suffered initially from poorly defined aims and objectives (*see* Chapter 5), which in turn reflected the inadequate planning of the clinic itself. In the future clinical protocols should be designed (*see* Chapter 6) and records that are 'audit friendly' used. This will make regular performance monitoring easier.

Case Study 2

Subject of audit

A process audit reviewing the efficiency of a screening programme for the 'over-75' population against the programme's objectives, using a proforma to collect data.

Background

Several years ago a practice decided to screen its elderly patients. The practice team met several times to review the available literature, after which it was agreed that the programme should assess primarily how the elderly functioned in their homes, rather than attempt to discover occult disease.

A standard proforma was used as a checklist for screening and also to facilitate the manual extraction of data at a later date. The 'at-risk' population was identified using the practice's age–sex register. It was divided into those who regularly attended the surgery, those who had regular home visits, either from a doctor, district nurse or health visitor, and those with whom the practice had had no recent contact.

Opportunistic screening was performed by the member of the practice team who made the next suitable contact. Patients who rarely attended were sent a standard letter outlining the purpose of the programme and were made an offer of an appointment at the surgery or a home visit.

Reason for audit

As opportunistic screening is time consuming it was important that an assessment should be made of the benefits to the elderly in relation to the effort involved.

Aims of audit

The audit was designed to:

- measure the uptake of the service by the target population
- assess/quantify the functional needs/deficits identified

- find out whether non-attenders had important unfulfilled needs
- assess the adequacy of the proforma.

Methods

The proforma was the primary data source. As the practice did not have a computer at that time, the proforma was structured in a form suitable for manual extraction by lay staff. A simple 'Yes/No' response format was used whenever possible, for example:

Hearing problem present	Yes/No
Hearing aid possessed	Yes/No
If Yes, hearing aid used	
etc.	

Who carried out the audit?

The data extraction and the subsequent analysis were carried out by one of the partners, who was particularly enthusiastic about the project, and the practice manager. However, the exercise could have been performed equally well by the administrative staff under the guidance of the practice manager, which would have been more cost-effective.

Results

As other surveys of this age group have shown, a variety of daily functional needs were revealed. Patients were identified who would benefit from hearing aids, spectacles, bath aids, meals on wheels, and so on. Data about dependency on others for help and recent bereavement were also obtained. A sample of some of the results is given in Table CS2.1.

The audit confirmed that the majority of people who make no demand on primary care, i.e. the group which did not seek medical advice regularly, had no major unmet needs. However, all the elderly patients questioned were positive in their attitude to the new service, and were impressed that their needs were being considered.

Table CS2.1   Elderly screening

Functional needs	%
Living alone	53
Depending on someone for help	56
Confined to home by ill health	36
Loss of someone close in last year	15
Concerned about current health	59
Recent visual problems	36
Recent hearing difficulties	27
Problems with bladder control	26

Changes resulting from audit

The resulting changes may be summarized as follows:

- As opportunistic screening gave the best yield, routine visits to people who were well were discontinued.
- The proforma was improved.
- An information sheet for patients was introduced.
- Subsequent reviews of results were to be carried out every three years.
- The practice manager and her staff were to organize and carry out subsequent reviews, as part of the regular monitoring of a service to patients.
- There would be a further exploration of patient attitudes to practice services (*see* Case Study 3).

Benefits of audit to the practice

- The practice team established what they were doing.
- The basis for subsequent improvement could be readily identified, and so the desirable changes were easy to institute.
- Patient satisfaction with the services was documented.
- The practice team felt reassured that they were developing a service of benefit and value to patients, and which was becoming cost-effective.

Comment

This is another simple practice activity analysis (*see* Chapter 7) which was well planned and with testable aims. It was seen as an integral part of managing this part of the practice's services.

Case Study 3

Subject of audit

AN audit of process and outcome, reviewing the impact of a screening service for the elderly on patient satisfaction. It used a self-administered patient questionnaire, and assessed whether screening and similar services would improve the practice's image with patients.

Background

A recent audit (Case study 2) by a practice team of the screening of its 'over-75' population had confirmed that, although most people who make no call on the practice services have no need of them, the elderly population were very positive about screening.

Reason for audit

A desire to find out more about the attitude of patients to planned preventive care offered by the practice, and to assess its effect on the practice image.

Aim of audit

To test the belief of the practice team that planned preventive services are welcomed by patients.

Method

The practice carried out a postal audit of patient satisfaction using a self-administered questionnaire with Likert scales. A representative sample of patients was drawn using the practice age–sex register. Results were collated and analysed by one partner and the practice manager.

An extract from the questionnaire is shown below.

The practice is developing new preventive services for patients. Our aim is to stop illness before it starts and so hopefully ensure healthier and happier patients. Could you spend a few minutes answering some questions?

1. Did you know about the following services provided at the surgery?

Well Women checks	Yes	No	Unsure
Well Man checks	Yes	No	Unsure
Elderly checks	Yes	No	Unsure
... etc.			

2. Which of the following services have you used?

Well Women checks	Yes	No	Unsure
Well Man checks	Yes	No	Unsure
Elderly checks	Yes	No	Unsure
... etc.			

3. If you have not used these services would you be likely to in the future?

Well Women checks	Yes	No	Unsure
Well Man checks	Yes	No	Unsure
Elderly checks	Yes	No	Unsure
... etc.			

4. Are there services we do not provide that you feel we should? Please comment if you wish.

5. In general I think the practice provides a good service.

1	2	3	4	5
strongly agree	agree	unsure	disagree	strongly disagree

6. The new preventive services are an improvement in the services of the practice.

1	2	3	4	5
strongly agree	agree	unsure	disagree	strongly disagree

7. The surgery hours are convenient to me.

1	2	3	4	5
strongly agree	agree	unsure	disagree	strongly disagree

Please comment if you wish.

8. I feel I could see a doctor today without an appointment if I felt I needed to.

1	2	3	4	5
strongly agree	agree	unsure	disagree	strongly disagree

and so on...

Results

The response rate varied by age. The elderly had the highest response rate, at about 90%. Men between the ages of 30 and 65 had the lowest response rate, at 65%.

The survey provided useful information about patients' views on the practice's services. In terms of preventive care, the results suggested that, overall, patients preferred targeted preventive clinics to opportunistic screening. Conversely, patients who made little use of the practice currently indicated that they would be unlikely to make use of planned preventive services in future; however, they tended to believe that the services offered were 'a good thing' and improved their view of the practice.

Changes resulting from the audit

The results of the audit:

- helped to shape new preventive services
- led to improvements in the practice leaflet
- prompted the practice to explore further how it might gather patients' opinions and suggestions for improvement on a regular basis.

Was the audit repeated?

No, it was considered unnecessary. However, further audits of patient satisfaction are planned, which will focus on patient uptake and use of regular services for the acutely and chronically ill.

Comment

The practice had decided to carry out this particular audit because the results of the first audit (Case Study 2) had suggested that the practice image was improved by the provision of a particular service. The practice team decided to verify this impression because it could have important consequences for practice policy.

In the past it was rare for doctors to carry out patient satisfaction surveys. It is important that such questionnaires are worded carefully to ensure that patients record what they really feel. In this particular case the questionnaire was sent to a representative sample of patients, but it could have given very useful information had it been administered to surgery attenders at the conclusion of a consultation.

Looking ahead, audits of patient satisfaction are likely to become increasingly important. Some surveys will be district wide, carried out by the health authority. Nevertheless, it is important for practices to assess patient satisfaction themselves on a regular sampling basis. Audits of patient satisfaction help a practice team to know whether its services are what patients want, and whether they are of an acceptable standard. They can be used as a tool to improve the practice image by showing that doctors care about their patients, and that they are prepared to respond to unmet needs.

Case Study 4

Subject of audit

A process audit attempting to reduce clinical error by comparing performance with a practice standard for the care of patients with epilepsy, using a records review.

Background

One of the advantages of having a registrar within a practice is that they can stimulate change. This particular practice had two registrars, who had carried out an audit of the care of patients with epilepsy in the practice. The outstanding finding for that audit was that over 50% of patients with epilepsy had not been seen by a doctor or nurse in the previous year.

As a result, the practice team formulated an explicit standard, incorporated in a protocol, requiring that every patient with epilepsy on medication should be reviewed at least once a year. The practice team expected that this would improve the consistency of its performance. This audit was designed to show whether the care showed an improvement, in terms of patient contacts, upon that revealed by the baseline audit.

Reason for audit

Despite having a basic standard, the practice's handling of patients with epilepsy still seemed to be variable.

Aim of audit

To assess the degree of compliance with the practice protocol.

Method

At the time of the audit the practice had a manual diagnostic index including the names of known patients with epilepsy. Using this, patient notes were identified and reviewed. While the notes were out, the opportunity was also taken to review the diagnosis and the appropriateness of treatment.

Who carried out the audit?

The records review was carried out by one of the partners who had a particular interest in epilepsy.

Results

Of the 54 patients, entered as suffering from epilepsy on the manual diagnostic index, the diagnosis was thought to be correct in 51 cases. Further results are given in Table CS4.1.

There had been no improvement in the contact rate with patients, and the practice criteria and standards were not being met. Further, the results raised more general questions about the functioning of the repeat prescription system.

Table CS4.1   Reason for patient contact in the last five years

Reason for contact	No. of contacts
A fit	13
Drug review	29
New patient contact	2
Initial diagnosis	4
No clear contact	3
Number seen *in last year*	25

Changes resulting from audit

The embarrassing findings of this audit stimulated a series of meetings within the practice. These resulted in:

• the construction of an internal clinical guideline for the management of epilepsy, and better protocols to try and ensure action on routine procedures

- an overhaul of the repeat prescribing systems
- a decision that partners should update their knowledge of epilepsy management.

Was the audit repeated?

The audit has not been repeated as yet. However, this is clearly an area where continuous audits will be required until the practice can be sure that its own standards are achieved and maintained. Future audits of the modified repeat prescription system are planned, to see if that works as intended.

Benefits to practice

- A better standard of care for patients with epilepsy.
- The prospect of improvement in the repeat prescription system.
- The need for new clinical knowledge and skills was identified.
- Improved professional satisfaction for the doctors and nurses involved in epilepsy care.

Comment

This audit demonstrates the value of having specific clinical criteria and standards against which subsequent care can be assessed (*see* Chapter 6). It is a reminder that having such criteria and standards is not of itself sufficient, because they are not always implemented by clinicians. Audit reveals the gap between intention and reality and in doing so becomes a powerful tool for ensuring implementation.

As in Case studies 2 and 3, the practice had management arrangements that enabled the changes identified as necessary to be implemented.

Case Study 5

Subject of audit

AN audit of process and intermediate outcome to improve the effectiveness of rubella immunization among adolescent girls within the practice population, using practice activity analysis.

Background

For many years the routine immunization of young women against rubella had been carried out by the medical and nursing staff of the health authority. The practice had identified certain problems arising from this.

1 Information about children immunized was often slow in arriving from the health authority, which meant that the practice records of those patients were incomplete.
2 Some girls were unsure whether they had been immunized.

It became clear that staffing problems at the clinic were causing delays in immunizing; immunization had become a crisis response by the authority to a request from the practice for information about the rubella status of individual patients. The practice team decided to take over the provision of this service, and the practice nurse was given responsibility for it.

Reason for audit

To ensure that the practice service was at least as effective as the local authority system.

Aims of audit

The aims were:

- to measure the immunization status of eligible females at eight months and two years after the installation of the new programme
- to provide feedback on effectiveness to the practice nurse and partners.

Method

Girls eligible for immunization were identified and sent for using the age–sex register. If a girl failed to respond to two requests, her mother was contacted by telephone and, if possible, the girl was offered another appointment or the reason for non-attendance was discovered and listed.

The practice nurse assessed the results, although it could have been done by any member of the administrative staff.

Results

The results are shown in Table CS5.1.

This audit showed a higher level of uptake in year one than in year two, but for both years the uptake was much higher than that achieved by the health authority. Fear of needles was given as the main reason for refusal.

Changes resulting from audit

The practice nurse had clear evidence of her effectiveness and the partners were satisfied that the new arrangements were better than immunization through the health authority clinic. No major changes were considered necessary. Nevertheless, the practice formulated a new target: to achieve a 100% immunization rate. The partners chose an ideal standard (*see* Chapter 6) because they recognized that effective protection is person specific. The practice nurse also sought new strategies to persuade defaulters to be immunized.

Table CS5.1   Comparative immunization notes

Action	Year 1 (at 8 months)	Year 2
Girls called	51	41
Immunized at surgery	45	36
Immunized at school	2	1
Refused	2	4
Agreed to have immunization later	2	0

Was the audit repeated?

With the advent of computerization in the practice, continuous performance monitoring became the operational practice. The immunization status of girls on the practice list is recorded in the practice nurse's annual report to the partnership: 100% rates are now achieved consistently year on year.

Comment

This audit shows the relationship between the process of care and its outcome in terms of protection against rubella conferred on patients at risk. It is one of the few situations where an 'ideal' standard is both clinically desirable and achievable, *provided* that the practice operates continuous performance monitoring, and therefore vigorous follow up of defaulters, as part of its management function.

Case Study 6

Subject of audit

A process audit attempting to reduce clinical error in the use of H_2-antagonists by case review.

Background

This partnership uses a practice formulary. It was agreed that the H_2-antagonist to be prescribed routinely should be cimetidine.

Reason for audit

PACT data had revealed more prescribing of ranitidine than was agreed by policy. The question was whether there was a noteworthy departure from the practice standard for the prescription of H_2-antagonists, and if so why.

Aim of audit

To review the prescribing patterns of cimetidine and ranitidine and to establish current practice.

Method

Patients on repeat prescriptions for either cimetidine or ranitidine were identified from the data held on the practice computer. In addition, any patient given a prescription for an H_2-antagonist during a consultation was noted.

The manual records of all patients were reviewed and the reasons for prescribing identified.

The objectives of the records review were:

- to determine the pattern of H_2-antagonist use
- to find out whether partners were complying with practice standards, which required that:
  (a) the preferred practice H_2-antagonist should be cimetidine
  (b) a clear diagnosis of peptic ulcer or hiatus hernia should be made before prescribing
  (c) all patients taking H_2-antagonists should be encouraged to take them episodically rather than permanently.

Who carried out the audit?

As clinical data were involved the records review was carried out by the partners; one partner had responsibility for ensuring that the task was completed, and for collating and analysing the data.

Results

In general, the partners felt that there was reasonable compliance with the practice standards. As an illustration, one partner had 25 patients taking cimetidine, 400 mg; of these, 25 had a proven diagnosis, seven took episodic treatment, four had never been tried off treatment, 13 had been off treatment but without long-term success, and one had just started treatment.

Another partner had 19 patients taking ranitidine, 150 mg; of these, 16 had a clear diagnosis, six took episodic treatment, eight had never been tried off long-term treatment, four had been tried off long-term but without long-term effect, and one had died of unrelated illness.

Personal analyses were available for all partners, which could be compared with aggregated results.

Changes resulting from audit

At a clinical meeting to discuss the results, it was decided that:

- it was not necessary to change the formulary
- the notes of patients who had not been tried off treatment should be tagged, so that there would be an opportunity to consider episodic treatment in future with their doctor
- the objective of removing some patients from the hospital follow-up clinics should be pursued.

Was the audit repeated?

Future audits will be performed to check that the standard is still being followed, as part of a regular review of PACT data. Patients attending hospitals for dyspeptic symptoms, and the reasons for them, have been the subject of consequential audit.

Comment

This audit highlighted the amount of work involved in the manual analysis of notes (*see* Chapter 7). If this type of audit is to become routine, partners must train non-medical staff to undertake it.

The audit demonstrated that the discussion and analysis by the partners was inadequate. Although confronted with personal and aggregate data showing apparently significant divergences from their own explicit criteria and standards, they chose to pass over these. This pattern of behaviour can easily go unquestioned unless the practice has an effective system for handling the results of audit and bringing about change (*see* Chapter 10).

Case Study 7

Subject of audit

A process audit demonstrating the standard of care in the practice through the use of a tracer condition, namely hypertension.

Background

About ten years ago a practice team decided to audit its care of patients with hypertension, after which it introduced some explicit criteria for care. The questions considered by the partners were as follows:

- We believe we provide good care for our patients with hypertension. Is that true?
- What standards can be measured?
- Do these provide evidence of good care?
- How does our care compare with defined standards?
- How does my care compare with that of my partners/my peers?
- Can I improve?
- Should I improve?

The original criteria and standards for the care of hypertensives as agreed by the practice are listed below.

- The initial diagnosis should be based on three (minimum) recordings of a diastolic pressure > 100 mmHg.
- There should be a record of:
  - urine analysis
  - smoking history
  - family history
  - height and weight.
- The medication should be recorded.
- The current (controlled) diastolic pressure should be < 90 mmHg and should be recorded within the preceding year.

Reason for the audit

A new registrar commented to the partners that she could not reconcile the practice's stated belief that it provided good care for its hypertensive patients with her difficulty in finding information in the notes. The second reason for audit was the death of a 62-year-old man from a cerebrovascular accident who, when the notes were examined, had had a diagnosis of hypertension some 15 years previously. This had been treated for about five years and then was lost to follow-up, although there were several entries in the notes about other consultations. These incidents led the practice team to question its perception of hypertensive care and to audit its compliance with its own protocols.

Methods

The practice team decided to use hypertension as a tracer condition (*see* Chapter 8) to examine aspects of chronic care. The audit was carried out when the practice had no disease index or computer. Patients with hypertension were identified in three ways:

- when summarizing the clinical records in the practice
- from repeat prescriptions for antihypertensive drugs
- opportunistically in surgery and by the practice nurse.

With the cases identified the practice team drew up a simple data collection form which identified the year of diagnosis, smoking record, urine analysis and other characteristics in which the practice was interested. It was then just a relatively simple clerical task to go through the records and extract the information.

Results of the audit

The results of this audit were disturbing. Although the prevalence rate and the age–sex distribution of hypertension in the practice matched the figures expected, only 32% of patients had three prediagnostic diastolic blood pressure measurements taken. On average, smoking was recorded in 60% of patients but there were wide variations among partners in recording; urine analysis was recorded in < 50% of cases, family history in < 15%, height in < 10% and weight in < 15%. Current medication was recorded in 98% of cases, and 80% had a recent diastolic pressure of < 90 mmHg.

The partners felt that, if their diagnosis had been correct originally, the treatment they were prescribing was reasonably successful. However, this audit did not demonstrate good care as they had previously defined it. It was also obvious that the clinical record-keeping was incomplete.

Changes resulting from audit

Discussion of the results led to the following changes:

- Revision of the protocol to include, for example, the measurement of fasting lipids, and an agreement about the drugs to prescribe for hypertension.
- Acceptance of a protocol for the diagnosis and management of patients with hypertension.
- An agreement about what to record.
- The development of a vascular clinic where the practice nurse works to a protocol generated by the doctors.
- Definition of the role of the team in measuring, recording and advising on hypertension.

Was the audit repeated?

A repeat audit has demonstrated that 100% of the hypertensive patients have their smoking and urine analysis recorded, 90% have family history recorded, and 100% have their weight and height recorded. Since the generation of the protocol, all new diagnoses have been based on three diastolic pressure measurements of > 100 mmHg.

Postscript

Since 1990, when this audit was first described, there have been many changes in the way the practice works. Much of this change relates to computerization. Changes in the GP contract relating to producing statistics for targets have also had some impact. Audit is now part of the practice routine. All records are now on computer and the data that previously had to be extracted manually in a painstaking way are easily available. The practice now only uses the paper records for filing reports and letters. Data are entered by all the team during consultations or from reports from hospitals or other agencies. The information is audited routinely by the computer manager and the audit data are fed back to the team regularly.

The standards to be achieved for clinical conditions such as hypertension are now reviewed annually by the practice, and incorporate changes in guidelines from such organizations as the British Hypertension Society,[1] where the practice feels these are appropriate.

The majority of the management of hypertension is carried out by the practice nursing staff, working to an agreed protocol, recording data on to the computer and using the call and recall system for follow-up.

Since the original report, the practice protocol has expanded to include:

- treatment of systolic hypertension
- measurement of cholesterol and lipids, and treatment where appropriate
- recording of 'non-drug' treatment.

Confidence in the data has given the practice the ability to determine the quality of its management of hypertension, and to start linking the quality with morbidity outcomes.

Lastly, this series of audits also stimulated the practice team to examine its clinical care in two other areas – asthma and gout. The audit of the treatment of patients with gout showed reasonable doctor compliance with the practice's predetermined standard for the frequency of checking and the target serum level of uric acid to be achieved. However, there were major inter-partner differences in the treatment of asthmatic patients, for example in the use of peak flow recordings and the number of different drugs prescribed. These variations reflected the fact that the practice had no agreed protocols or standards for the treatment of asthma, and consequently the quality of the medical record-keeping was also variable.

Revised protocols for asthma and gout are now in use, and patients with these conditions are subject to further regular monitoring to ensure partner compliance with agreed protocols and standards.

Comment

All those involved in health care may have a different perception of good care. Audit can be used to demonstrate different things for different people: to a politician it will have to measure cost-effectiveness; to a manager it will have to measure efficiency; to a receptionist possibly punctuality; to a doctor job satisfaction; to a patient, concern, interest, and relief from the illness.

For most audit processes, demonstrating good care often starts with simple questions. In this case, did all patients with a diagnosis of hypertension have a blood pressure recording in the notes in the last year? The pattern of recording data was not originally compatible with good care: there were demonstrable gaps in performance when compared with agreed standards. An improvement in record-keeping was necessary and, as a result, good care and control can now be demonstrated to patients by using computer graphics, computer protocols and checklists. These also remind partners of the standards previously agreed. An improvement in morbidity or mortality has yet to be demonstrated.

The case study also demonstrates that the stimulus of the results generated by the initial audit led to a cyclical process of improvement and refinement over time of quite striking proportions. Throughout, the practice team retained full control because they were able to see, through continuous performance monitoring, exactly where they had got to in their development at any particular point in time.

Case Study 8

Subject of audit

A review of organizational error to establish why supposed improvements in the quality of management within a practice through the appointment of a deputy practice manager had not achieved the desired results (*see* Chapter 10).

Background

The experience, education and reading of the partners had convinced them that good management at the doctor–patient level normally led to an improvement in clinical care and an increase in job satisfaction.[1,2] They believed that improved management in the wider context should result in improvements to the functioning of the partnership, and ultimately to better services for patients.[3]

A practice manager was appointed in 1983, in response to an increasingly complex administrative burden. The person appointed was computer literate, the ex-personnel manager of a large hotel, who also ran the financial side of a small business. The new manager was left to develop the practice and her own role within it.

Five years later, the size and complexity of the practice had increased. Consequently, the practice manager had become increasingly busy. She had attended several courses on practice management and was anxious to extend her role in the development of the practice and its quality of care. To achieve these objectives, she proposed to the partners that a deputy practice manager be appointed to take over the routine administration of the practice, so that she could be released to obtain further training through an Open University course, and participate more in the strategic management of the practice.

A deputy practice manager was appointed, who had experience of managing people and finance.

Reason for the audit

Initially the new appointment seemed to work well. However, the practice manager became busier. She was still administering the practice, trying to teach the deputy, and the course work was beginning to arrive in quantity. Unfortunately, three months after the appointment of the deputy the practice manager went on sick leave with a disabling physical condition.

The partners turned to the deputy practice manager to take over. However, it became apparent that the practice manager was the only person who knew how to run the practice. The partners realized that having a deputy practice manager did not ensure continuity of quality of management, nor did it provide the enhanced management input that they had expected. They decided to identify the main organizational areas of the practice and delegate them to specific partners, who would have the power to make an executive decision in each area.

The partners met regularly to make management decisions on behalf of the absent practice manager, and it was decided that this approach would be more efficient than unstructured management meetings. It mirrored the way the partners had dealt with clinical policy decisions for years: one partner delegated to research a particular clinical area brought his or her ideas for discussion with the other partners, to agree a clinical protocol that had been devised after appropriate discussion.

The deputy practice manager returned to her previous job. The partners took the opportunity to investigate whether the post of deputy practice manager could help improve the quality of practice management.

Aim of the audit

To review the existing management structure and to assess it against the management needs of the practice.

Method

The original aims of appointing a deputy practice manager were re-examined and a chart showing the current organization was drawn up. The roles played by the partners, the practice manager and the other staff in the decision to appoint a deputy practice manager were also examined.

Who carried out the audit?

Owing to the fundamental nature of the audit, it was undertaken by all partners with the support of the existing practice manager.

Results

The basic finding was that the responsibilities of the deputy practice manager had not been thought about by anyone other than the practice manager. Each of the partners and staff members had different perceptions of the role of the deputy and of the practice manager herself.

It was also clear that the partnership's decision-making process was inadequate: a considerable amount of the practice manager's time was spent on trying to obtain appropriate decisions. Either the practice manager made decisions on her own, or was forced to present issues to all of the partners, which took time. Initially, the partners had not delegated to each other responsibility for particular parts of practice organization; this would have given the practice manager points of reference and helped the decision-making process. It would then have been possible to identify the range of decisions that could be made by the practice manager alone, by the practice manager and the relevant partner, and by the whole partnership

The problems that led to failure to achieve the stated objectives in appointing a deputy practice manager were as follows:

- poor communication and decision-making mechanisms at partnership level

- inexperience and poor training of the deputy practice manager in the practical aspects of the functioning of the practice
- the demography of the practice – two large health centres caused duplication of effort in the implementation of policies
- unrealistic expectations of the deputy practice manager post among staff and partners.

Changes resulting from audit

Areas of activity

Key areas of practice managerial activity were identified as follows:

- Access and communication
- Buildings
- Education
- Emergencies and out of hours
- Equipment and computers
- Finance and fundholding
- Prescribing
- Preventive care
- Referral patterns
- Staff recruitment and training
- Teamwork and extracurricular activities
- The Contract.

These areas were assigned to various of the partners, who each had the executive power to make a decision in that area on behalf of the partnership while regularly reporting to the partnership on progress.

Two of the existing practice secretaries had applied for the post of deputy practice manager, having been on a local AMSPAR course. It was proposed to appoint them as office managers, one at each health centre. By splitting their existing jobs and appointing part-time secretaries to fill the secretarial gaps left by their redeployment, the practice was able to present the changes to the health authority as a no-cost option, while staffing levels remained unchanged. This strategy ensured that both office managers had experience and knowledge of the functioning of the practice. The agreed list of management areas within the practice was divided between the office managers, and it was clear which partner to consult in case of problems and which office manager. All were encouraged to share, so that absence did not mean the practice would be without effective management. The new management structure is shown in Fig. CS8.1.

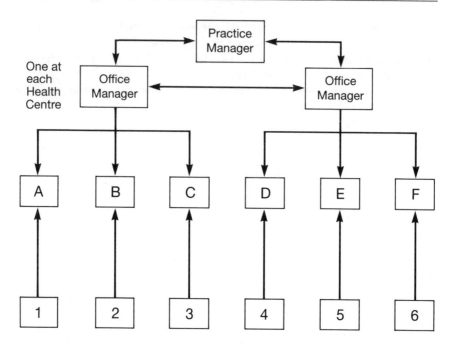

Key

A Teamwork/Communication
B Finance/Fundholding/Referrals
C Equipment/Computers/Out of Hours
D The Contract/Preventative Care
E Education(GP registrar)/Prescribing
F Staff/Buildings

The partners are represented by the numbers 1–6

Figure CS8.1 The new management structure

Development plan

When the practice manager returned to work her first task was to help the partners produce a plan for the further development of the practice through fundholding. This she was able to do because the responsibility for daily operational management had been delegated to the office managers and the relevant partners. She discussed these plans at length with the relevant partners, particularly those responsible for fundholding and staff, and the two office managers. They quickly identified all potential problems with regard to space, staff rotas and the long-term relationship between the fundholding staff and permanent staff. Appropriate appointments were made in record time.

Practice management

The benefits of the practice manager's Open University course also became apparent. The practice manager and office managers began to meet weekly to plan and implement office policies. Staff training assumed a higher priority, and staff were enrolled in local training courses. Delegation was encouraged, and staff were involved in solving their own problems rather than presenting the practice manager with a series of complaints. Each member of staff was offered a new contract, with better job definitions. The use of information technology within the practice began to improve.

Was the audit repeated?

As fundholding became established within the practice, more and more of the practice manager's time was taken up with this activity. Many tasks linked to fundholding tasks became routine. The day-to-day running of fundholding was beginning to get in the way of strategic management. An opportunity arose to employ a dedicated fund manager when hours were released by the two office managers expressing a wish to work part-time, owing to family commitments.

The practice manager found that, having given the routine financial running of the practice to an office manager, she was constantly having to update herself on the practice's financial position in order to manage the long-term business plan. This involved duplication of effort between the practice manager and the relevant office manager. With reduced hours the office manager dealing with practice finances handed this work back, thereby ceasing the duplication of effort.

When two partners retired the new partnership developed a mission statement: 'the practice will deliver the highest possible standard of care to its patients, while considering the physical, mental and financial health of the partners and staff', and the clinical care that the practice was delivering came under close scrutiny. The delivery of this mission statement was dependent on fundholding strategy, and a strong management structure was seen to be increasingly important.

When the management structure was reaudited the issues raised above were addressed. Regular reviews of overall strategy had been effected by the practice manager and one partner cooperating closely and meeting regularly to discuss management issues. This had greatly facilitated management decisions within the partnership. Two of the partners now give direct support to the practice manager in the areas of financial and strategic planning, a fund manager has been appointed, the office managers now work effectively on a part-time basis, and the executive roles of the partners have been redistributed.

These latest developments are shown in Fig. CS8.2.

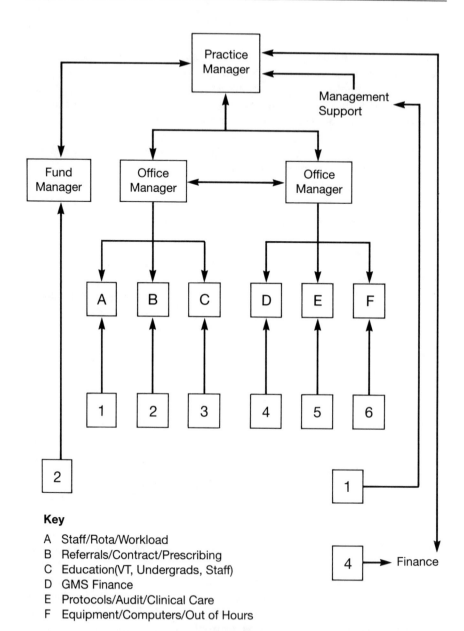

Key

A Staff/Rota/Workload
B Referrals/Contract/Prescribing
C Education(VT, Undergrads, Staff)
D GMS Finance
E Protocols/Audit/Clinical Care
F Equipment/Computers/Out of Hours

The partners are represented by the numbers 1–6

Figure CS8.2 The latest management structure

Comment

By tracing the contributing factors to a management action by the partners, this audit revealed not only whether the desired end had been achieved (which it had not), but also whether the management processes were effective. Audit allowed the identification of an organizational error, i.e. the appointment of a deputy practice manager, and alternative solutions could be introduced once the problem had been evaluated.

The repetition of the audit cycle (i.e. a further review of the existing management structure and its assessment against the needs of the practice) led to a further refinement of the management structure of the practice, which enabled it to cope with new needs and developments. This case study demonstrates how effective an audit of process can be in changing organizations.

Case Study 9

Subject of audit

AN audit of high-risk hypertensive patients in a practice of five partners and 10 500 patients.

Background

The British Hypertension Society (BHS) recently published clinical guidelines that set standards for the treatment of hypertension[1] and these were adopted by the practice. The guidelines were particularly welcome, as for the first time they identified levels of systolic hypertension which warrant treatment and distinguished different categories of hypertensives who are most at risk of developing the complications of hypertension. It has been known for some time that hypertension is only one of several risk factors which contribute to an individual's chance of myocardial infarction (MI) or stroke, the others being cigarette smoking, diabetes, raised cholesterol, left ventricular hypertrophy (LVH), previous MI/stroke or cardiovascular event. These risk factors, if present in addition to hypertension, are not merely

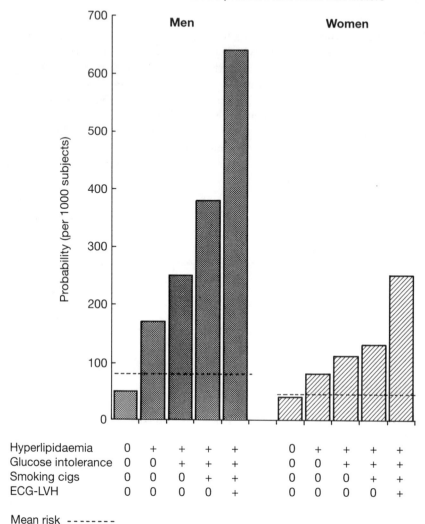

MORTALITY : Blood pressure and other risk factors

Hyperlipidaemia	0	+	+	+	+	0	+	+	+	+
Glucose intolerance	0	0	+	+	+	0	0	+	+	+
Smoking cigs	0	0	0	+	+	0	0	0	+	+
ECG-LVH	0	0	0	0	+	0	0	0	0	+

Mean risk - - - - - - - -

Figure CS9.1 To show how additional risk factors in addition to hypertension multiply the risk of mortality in hypertensives

additive, but tend to multiply an individual's risk of developing a fatal MI or stroke.[2] This is demonstrated in Fig. CS9.1.

Figure CS9.2 shows that lowering blood pressure, particularly in those who have two or more risk factors in addition to hypertension, would be especially beneficial. Reducing systolic pressure by 30 mmHg in a high-risk individual can reduce the probability of developing coronary heart disease

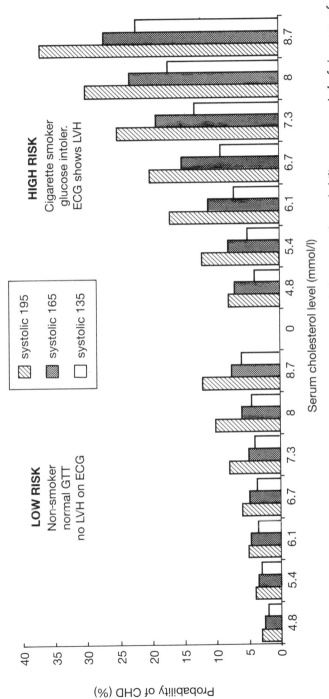

Figure CS9.2 To show the relationship between blood pressure ansd other risk factors on the probability, over a period of six years, of developing coronary heart disease (the lower the systolic BP, with any combination of risk factors, the lower the probability)

by a factor of 11%, whereas the same reduction in a low-risk individual will result in only a 1% reduction in risk. The BHS suggests that a suitable level of blood pressure control for all hypertensives should be 160 mmHg systolic or below and 90 mmHg diastolic or below, but examination of Fig. CS9.2 shows that an individual's risk continues to fall as the level of blood pressure is reduced, and the lower the values the better.

The elimination of smoking and the reduction of raised cholesterol is very difficult in practice, and the presence of LVH, diabetes or previous MI or stroke is immutable. The reduction of raised blood pressure is comparatively straightforward. The approach of concentrating therapeutic effort on a relatively small number of high-risk patients has been advocated by others.[3]

Aims of audit

To identify all hypertensive patients in the practice who have two or more risk factors for cardiovascular disease in addition to their hypertension, and to show whether their blood pressure is well controlled.

The standard

All patients identified with two or more risk factors in addition to hypertension should have their blood pressure reduced to 150 mmHg systolic or below, and their diastolic to 80 mmHg or below.

Data collection

Sixty-nine patients were identified with two or more risk factors out of a total of 949 hypertensives.

The data were difficult to find. A systematic approach to the management of hypertension was adopted by the practice in 1987. At that time, cholesterol was not routinely measured in all hypertensives. In 1992 the practice criteria changed to include cholesterol measurement in hypertensives, but not all those diagnosed and being treated before 1992 had subsequently had a cholesterol measurement.

Despite having had a computer capable of handling hypertensive data since 1987, not all the relevant data (particularly 'old' cholesterol measurements and smoking status) had been computerized. A hand search of the 949 notes of those patients with hypertension was undertaken, and a grant of £250 from the local MAAG to undertake this task was appreciated.

As the notes were examined, those without relevant recordings of all risk factors were tagged in an attempt to improve the numbers of patients with hypertension with all risk factors recorded (this effort formed the basis of another audit).

Comparison of target population with the standard

Sixty of the 69 patients in the audit had a blood pressure at the end of the first data collection which was above 150 mmHg systolic and 80 mmHg diastolic. This is shown in Table CS9.1, which also shows how the separate systolic and diastolic blood pressures of the audit group of patients matched the standard at the start of the audit. Table CS9.2 shows the relevant breakdown of the other risk factors in addition to hypertension in the audit group.

Implementation of change

The practice took four initiatives to improve the control of hypertension in patients with two or more risk factors.

Table CS9.1 The number of patients (%) with a blood pressure matching the standard at the beginning of the audit cycle

$n = 69$	Blood pressure reading		
	Systolic ≤ 150	Diastolic ≤ 80	Systolic/diastolic ≤ 150/80
Number of patients	24	19	9
(%)	(35)	(28)	(13)

Table CS9.2 Risk factors for cardiovascular disease, in addition to hypertension, in the audit group of patients

$n = 69$	Other risk factors associated with cardiovascular disease			
	Diabetes	Cholesterol >6.5	Smoking	End-organ damage*
Number of patients	32	35	27	53
(%)	(46)	(51)	(39)	(77)

*End-organ damage means ischaemic heart disease, stroke, transient ischaemic attack, peripheral vascular disease or ECG changes of left ventricular hypertrophy

1 A new blood pressure record card was designed, printed and introduced. The new card clearly indicates on the front the number and type of risk factors the individual carries (completed in red if there are two or more risk factors), plus a box into which a red star is inserted if two or more risk factors are present. All data were transferred to a new blood pressure record card for the 69 patients who were the subjects of this audit. An example of the old and new record cards is shown in Appendices 1 and 2.

HYPERTENSION RECORD CARD

SURNAME   FORENAME(S)   M
                                                         S
                                                         W

ADDRESS

TELEPHONE NUMBER
DATE OF BIRTH
GP

CUFF SIZE   STANDARD/LARGE/THIGH
ARM   RIGHT/LEFT
POSITION   SITTING/STANDING/LYING

RISK FACTORS – SMOKER
                WEIGHT
                ALCOHOL
                OCCUPATION
Examinations and Test
                PHYSICAL
                RENAL FUNCTION
                CVS FUNCTION
                FUNDI

DATE OF ONSET

BP LIMITS

APPENDIX 1 Hypertension card used at Coquet Medical Group until the start of this audit

Coquet Medical Group
Hypertension Record Card

Name	Forename(s)	M S W

Address	☎
	GP

Date of birth:-	Date of onset:-
	BMI at onset:-
Cuff size:- 35cm / 52cm	Arm:- Right / Left

Risk factors	Date:-				
Smoking (no./day)					
Alcohol (units/week)					
Lipids (raised/normal)					
End-organ damage (yes/no)					

Circle no. of risk factors (plus Diabetes if applicable)   0 1 2 ③ 4 5

★ Star = 2 or more risk factors

Initial physical examination Date:-	Initial investigations Date:-
CVS Kidneys Fundoscopy ECG	Electrolytes Creatinine Cholesterol γgt
Drugs	MCV Urine
	BP limits ≤160/90 or 150/80

APPENDIX 2   New hypertension card showing star (at least two risk factors for cardiovascular disease in addition to hypertension)

2 During the notes search, the notes and/or the blood pressure computer entry were highlighted for those patients whose blood pressure did not meet the agreed standard.

3 A series of meetings was organized in the practice at which the BHS guidelines and the concept of the advantages of concentrating particular effort on those patients with two or more risk factors were introduced. All the personnel concerned with the management of hypertensive patients attended regularly.

4 Patients with two or more risk factors who were attending nurse monitoring clinics were returned to GP surgeries for review, and were only returned to the nurse clinics when their blood pressure met the agreed standard.

Data revisited

The actual number of patients with two or more risk factors is rising as more established hypertensives have all their risk factors identified and as more patients develop hypertension and are identified, but this audit is confined to the originally identified 69 patients.

Tables CS9.3 and CS9.4 show the effect of the audit activity on the audit population, namely the practice team has improved the care of hypertension in the patients with two or more risk factors. Figures CS9.2 and CS9.3 show the information on systolic and diastolic pressures in graphical form. There has been a downward trend in both systolic and diastolic blood pressures. The number of patients with both systolic and diastolic blood pressure in the 'standard' range has improved from 9 (13%) to 17 (25%).

Table CS9.3 Number of patients (%) with a blood pressure matching the standard at the end of the audit cycle

$n = 69$	Blood pressure reading		
	Systolic $\leqslant 150$	Diastolic $\leqslant 80$	Systolic/diastolic $\leqslant 150/80$
Number of patients	37	28	17
(%)	(54)	(41)	(25)

Table CS9.4 Number of patients (%) with a blood pressure matching the standard at the beginning and at the end of the audit

BP reading	Number of patients (%)	
	At the start of the audit	At the end of the audit
Systolic ⩽ 150	24 (35)	37 (54)
Diastolic ⩽ 80	19 (28)	28 (41)
Systolic/diastolic ⩽ 150/80	9 13)	17 (25)

The future

All audits show that there is room for improvement. The practice has appointed a nurse practitioner who has a particular remit to audit the major chronic diseases of general practice, i.e. asthma, diabetes, hypertension, and cervical and breast cancer. It will be a specific part of her remit to keep the hypertensives with two or more risk factors under regular review, and to bring to the attention of the doctor and nurse responsible for the monitoring of these high-risk patients their current level of control, and to continue to flag notes and computer screens to act as an *aide-mémoire*.

Lessons

1 In a large practice one person should have specific responsibility for hypertension and its overall management.
2 The development, agreement and communication of guidelines across the practice takes patience.
3 Implementation of guidelines moves at different rates for different people in the team. It needs constant review and renewal of enthusiasm.
4 The treatment of hypertension, especially with the modern concepts of drug substitution rather than addition, is time consuming.
5 The drugs available for the treatment of hypertension, especially when there is a target of 150/80, are not ideal.
6 As each set of notes took approximately ten minutes to process from shelf to shelf, this work attracted a payment of approximately £1.50 an hour and was therefore only affordable if undertaken by a doctor and a nurse practitioner.

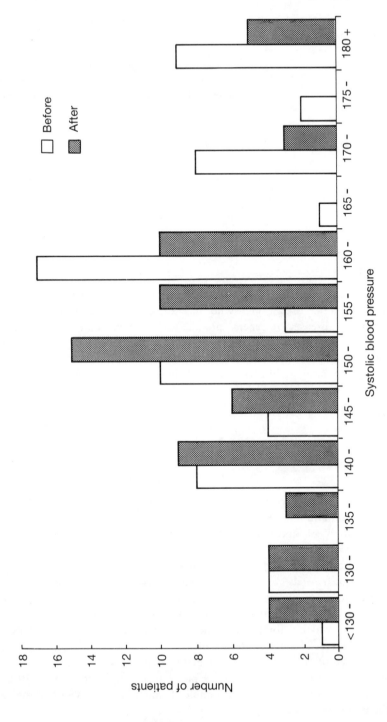

Figure CS9.3   To show the range in systolic blood pressures before and after the audit

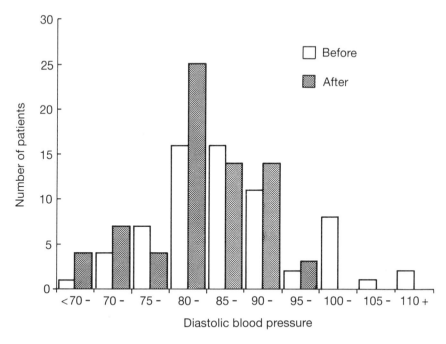

Figure CS9.4   To show the changes in diastolic blood pressure before and after the audit

Case Study 10

Subject of audit

To identify the reasons for frustration and irritation within a practice, and to enhance professional satisfaction.

Background

This practice comprised four partners (three male and one female); there were about 8500 patients registered, and the practice operated from a health authority clinic. The partners employed a senior receptionist/practice manager, a secretary, a part-time nurse and six part-time receptionists. A community nurse, a health visitor and a midwife were attached to the practice, but accountable to their own nursing hierarchies. The senior receptionist/practice manager had recently retired, and there was a new practice manager who had a commercial background, which was deemed important as the partners wanted to reappraise their management systems to ensure they met their own targets, maximized income and improved patient care.

Reason for the audit

The practice manager felt it was not possible for him to make any changes within the organization without a clear understanding of the reasons for the feelings of frustration, irritation and low morale exhibited by the practice team.

Aims of audit

To identify the reasons for the malaise within the practice, and to offer a range of solutions.

Methods

1 *Practice activity analysis*. The practice manager set up systems for collective data on attendance at surgeries and clinics, recording home visits and carrying out random checks comparing times of appointment against time patients were actually seen, by partner or by nurse.

   The partners looked at health authority returns on cervical cytology and preschool immunizations, and the practice manager assessed the availability of information on the rubella status of females in the practice, the monitoring of hypertension, and the over-75s screening programme.

2 *Patient satisfaction survey*. A survey of patient satisfaction was carried out after each consultation and consisted of a simple questionnaire (*see* Fig. CS10.1).

3 *A confidential enquiry to each member of staff*. They had to write a brief description of their job as they understood it to be, including all

1. These questions relate specifically to the consultation that you have just had.
   (i)   Did you see the doctor of your preferred choice?
         Yes/No
   (ii) Were you able to make this appointment for a time that suited you?
         Yes/No
   (iii) The length of time the consultation lasted was:
         (a) Too short to allow me to explain my problem.
   or   (b) Reasonable but I would have preferred longer.
   or   (c) About right.
   (iv) Were you seen promptly on your appointment time?
         Yes/No
   If your answer is No, then please answer the next questions:
   (v)   Did you have to wait up to 10 minutes?
         Did you have to wait more than 15 minutes?
         Did you have to wait more than 30 minutes?

The last question relates to the service the practice provides:
2. Overall, are you satisfied with the care and attention you get from the doctors and staff in the practice?
Yes/No/Don't know

Figure CS10.1   Patient survey

the tasks they were expected to do, describe (in absolute confidence) things that made the job more difficult than it need be, and identify any further training needs and what training they would like the practice to provide.

Who carried out the audit?

The audit was largely carried out under the direction of the practice manager, who was released from other duties for three months. Reception staff collected most of the data, and the partners encouraged patients to fill in the patient satisfaction survey.

Results

1 *Practice activity analysis.* An extract from data on consultation and hospital referral patterns, as part of the practice activity analysis, is shown in Table CS10.1. An extract from the immunization data collected is shown in Table CS10.2.

Table CS10.1 Consultation and referral rate

Doctor	Total surgery consultations	Doctor initiated consultations (%)	Extras (unlisted) (%)	Total home visits	Repeat visits (%)	'Clinic' consultations	Total patients seen	No. hospital referrals
Dr A	1241	36	10	256	27	349	1846	30
Dr B	1302	33	9	378	32	–	1680	36
Dr C	1291	25	12	357	19	323	1651	58
Dr D	1309	36	12	257	25	–	1566	34
Total	5143			1248		672	7063	158

Quarter 1 July–30 September
Consultation rate = 3.2
Referral rate = 75 per 1000 patients/year

Table CS10.2 Immunization rates

Children aged 2 years or under on the 1st of the (relevant) quarter.
Group I: Diphtheria, tetanus and polio (3 doses)
    78% of target population

Group II: Pertussis (3 doses)
    45% of target population

Group III: Measles (1 dose)
        or MMR
    69 of target population
NB: The local authority clinic had carried out 70% of these completed courses.

Children aged 5 years on 1st of the (relevant) quarter.
Preschool booster targets.
    76% of target population.
NB: The local authority clinic had carried out 95% of these.

Hypertension/smoking recording. Despite a declared policy of measuring blood pressure in all patients in the 40–65 years age group at least every five years, a random survey of one in ten records from the survey population showed that less than 50% had had their blood pressure recorded. The results were similar when the recording of smoking habit was examined: less than 50% of the records surveyed did not indicate whether the patient smoked.

2 *Patient satisfaction survey.* The results confirmed the suspicions of the practice that their poor time-keeping and inadequate appointment system were having an adverse effect on their relationships with their patients. However, the results from the general satisfaction question were encouraging and showed that the practice still had a positive image.

3 *Staff enquiry.* Information from the enquiry and interviews with the staff showed that the practice was not employing its full quota of reimbursable staff. The practice nurse felt she had neither the time nor the skills to make an appropriate contribution to the work of the practice. The employed staff had not been informed or consulted about any changes that were taking place; in particular, they felt threatened by the appointment of the practice manager.

In more general terms, the following deficiencies were identified in the practice:

- There was no common goal or purpose.
- There were no clinical protocols.
- The organization of the practice was inappropriate.
- There were no appraisals of performance.

- There was no recognition of training needs, nor any provision for meeting them.
- There was a dearth of good basic data regularly available.

Changes resulting from audit

The changes can be summarized as follows:

1 The practice started to have regular meetings, with an agenda and minutes.
2 The partners began to develop an agreed and written common purpose or goal.
3 The organizational structure of the practice was reviewed.
4 A clear definition of the relationships and responsibilities within the practice, particularly those between the practice manager and the doctors, was agreed.
5 Staff appraisals were introduced, based on new and agreed job descriptions.
6 A training programme for doctors and staff was set up: priority and resources were set aside for skills training for the practice nurse, and management training for one of the partners.
7 A series of practice meetings was instituted to discuss the production of clinical protocols.
8 The staff complement was increased.
9 More time was allocated for surgery and individual consultations.

Was the audit repeated?

This overall audit was not repeated, but a series of more specific audits were instituted to ensure that the practice team achieves its objectives in the key areas identified.

Comment

This case study demonstrated how an audit can be used to discover what is creating the frustration, irritation and inefficiency in a practice. Such an audit can be achieved only by the injection of a new resource: in this case, the new practice manager was given three months to investigate the problem, without which an external consultant would probably have had to be employed to identify the solutions.

Case Study 11

Subject of audit

A process audit to reduce clinical and organizational error, using the confidential case enquiry method.

Background

Mr and Mrs Black, their son Kevin (aged five years) and daughter Tracey (aged one year), had originally registered with the practice two years ago. Mr Black had been a labourer until recently, but was now out of work. Mrs Black was a nurse.

All the Blacks had active medical problems. Mr Black had chronic asthma, a condition for which he consulted Dr Adam regularly. Mrs Black had a long-standing history of undiagnosed, episodic abdominal pain, complicated by bouts of vomiting, especially in the evenings. She had seen Dr Baker regularly but, despite extensive investigation, no firm diagnosis had been established. When bouts of vomiting occurred the only intervention that gave reasonably prompt and symptomatic relief was intramuscular metocloparomide. Kevin was subject to recurrent earache and had recently had grommets inserted. Tracey had recently been diagnosed as suffering from an allergy to cow's milk. When the children became ill, Mrs Black tended to take them to see the doctor most readily available.

One evening, Kevin had a further attack of earache and Dr Edwards visited him at home. Dr Edwards found no serious abnormality and advised no medication. Kevin appeared comfortable.

The following day, Mr and Mrs Black took Kevin to hospital for a check-up on the grommets. They were told that one eardrum was inflamed, and that an antibiotic was indicated. Later that day, Mrs Black attended surgery with Tracey, when she saw Dr Collins. She asked Dr Collins how she could make a complaint about Dr Edwards who, she said, had failed to prescribe an antibiotic when the hospital doctor had said it was necessary. Dr Collins told Dr Edwards of the problem.

Reason for the audit

Dr Edwards was somewhat surprised by the complaint, because he had judged the child to be only slightly unwell and, as far as he could learn from Dr Baker, that was still the case. He decided to follow up the complaint with the parents, to see if he could find out what the problem really was, what seemed to have gone wrong, and to try and restore relationships.

He visited the parents, and during the course of the discussion (*see* below) it became clear that a more detailed enquiry, involving the management of all the members of the family, would be appropriate, i.e. a confidential, case-based audit was indicated.

Aims of audit

The purpose of the case audit was to define the family's concerns with particular regard to alleged clinical mismanagement. It would also try and establish what the family expected of the practice.

Method

In this confidential case enquiry, the following steps were taken:

1 An interview with the complainants.
2 A review of the case notes.
3 Recording the findings.
4 Discussion of the findings, leading to conclusions, with partners and patients (separately).

Who carried out the audit?

The audit was carried out by Dr Edwards as a continuation of his initial visit.

Results

The interview with the patients took just over one hour. The principal findings of fact were as follows:

1 The family had moved to this practice because of dissatisfaction with their previous practice. They were dismayed to find that in some respects the care they had received in this practice had not been of the standard they had expected.

2 Mr and Mrs Black thought that Dr Edwards, who had attended Kevin promptly, had been cursory in his examination and brief in his discussion of the problem.

3 Mrs Black was unhappy about the treatment she received for her sickness and abdominal pain when symptoms presented out of hours, and when a partner other than Dr Baker came: 'I'm never right until I get some Maxolon, and I shouldn't have to say that every time', she said. Nevertheless, she liked Dr Baker, had confidence in her, and wished only that there could be better communication between Dr Baker and the other partners about the management of Mrs Black in an emergency.

4 Both parents thought that Dr Collins should have diagnosed Tracey's milk allergy sooner.

5 Mr Black said that he was very satisfied with Dr Adam's treatment of his asthma.

6 There seemed to be no good reason, other than parental convenience, why the children tended to be taken to any partner, rather than the partner with whom the child was registered.

Mr Black, commenting on the practice, said that in the main he and his wife were satisfied with their care but they were surprised that the care could easily become less satisfactory in patches: 'Surely you must have some systems for dealing with families like us who have more than one problem on the go at once'.

The essential findings from this interview were passed to the other partners. The second stage of the audit began with a review of the case notes of all the family members. The case notes describing the management of both Mr and Mrs Black were considered to be full and appropriate, each giving a coherent account of their problems, the working diagnoses and the management plans, including up-to-date drug treatment. The case notes for the children were more brief, revealed multiple partner entries, and underlined the parent's impression of discontinuity leading, in Tracey's case, to delay in diagnosis, and, in Kevin's case, to conflicting advice on the management of the ear condition.

In the opinion of the partners, the interview and case notes review had shown that the parents' initial complaint about Dr Edwards was a token presentation of an underlying problem, rather than a reflection of a serious single error. Seen in that way, the complaint was basically justified. Problems of continuity and communication were revealed that reflected deficiencies in the practice's systems, and therefore such problems could recur.

Changes resulting form audit

Changes were grouped under three main headings.

1 *For the Black family.* To improve continuity of care for the children, Mr and Mrs Black agreed with the partners on the following:
   - Both children would be reregistered with Dr Baker. When Dr Baker was unavailable, the first alternative would be Dr Adam.
   - All partners were fully briefed by Dr Baker on Mrs Black's problem with abdominal pain, and how best to manage it.
   - The focus on two doctors for the family (rather than one, which might have been considered ideal) reflected the desire of both Mr Black and Mrs Black to keep their 'own doctor', that is Dr Adam and Dr Baker.

2 *Impact on practice systems.* The case raised several questions about practice systems, especially those bearing on continuity. These are now being considered further by the practice manager, and supplementary audits may be performed.

3 *For the audit procedure.* The case prompted further discussion among the partners about the value of auditing significant events. Two points were made. The question of who should be responsible for such audits was raised. In this instance, the benefits of the person about whom the complaint had been made were traded against the potential lack of objectivity which could result through personal involvement. There seemed to be no easy answer. In principle, it was felt that an uninvolved partner would be best placed to conduct such enquiries whenever possible.

   Second, the method should have included formal interviews with the partners concerned about their particular contributions to the family's care; ideally, this should have involved the relevant hospital doctors.

Comment

It is often said that an effective audit cannot be carried out on one case. However, this case study illustrates that this is untrue if the yardstick is to be change resulting in an improvement in care both for the individual patient and more generally. Significant event audits represent excellent value for money, in that the circumstances that provoke them are likely to result in change. There are no complicated data to collect, no difficult analyses to be made, and no expense to be incurred other than the time and care involved in the examination itself.

Confidential case enquiries are threatening because they involve an exploration of probable error. It is unlikely that the partners in this case would have consented to this kind of audit unless there had been prior agreement that such a method would be used, and that the results would be kept confidential within the practice. This case study helps to illustrate the general points about the handling of confidential case enquiries described in Chapter 8.

Case Study 12

Subject of audit

AUDIT of process and outcome assessing the effectiveness of a changed approach to the delivery of diabetes care.

Background

In 1985, a practice was concerned about its delivery of diabetes care. It was decided to set up a diabetes clinic, to identify and register all diagnosed diabetic patients and provide a framework of care for those not attending hospital clinics.

The practice compiled a diabetes register, produced a clinical guideline and operational protocols for care, established a team for diabetes care and identified the roles of the members of the team – the practice nurse was given lead responsibility.

Reason for the audit

After four years' experience, the practice team recognized that they had never tested whether the setting up of the diabetes clinic had led to improved patient care. Considerably more resources were being put into the management of this particular condition, with no evidence to show that patient care had improved. Hence the 1989 audit, but the process of periodic review did not stop there. Hence the further audits carried out in 1991 and 1995.

Aims of audit

To test whether the establishment of the diabetes clinic had led to improved patient care, in terms of improved patient education about the condition, better control of the disease and the effective use of formal nursing input.

Method

As an audit-friendly format for patient records had been used from the outset, a simple record-based audit could be carried out. The following were regarded as essential for the recorded data:

- date the patient was last seen
- whether the patient received GP or hospital care
- whether the patient received insulin
- the patient's current drug therapy
- data and result of patient's last
  - eye test
  - foot examinations/advice/chiropody
  - blood pressure
  - weight/body mass index
  - urine analysis for proteins
  - glycosylated protein estimation.

Who carried out the audit?

The audit was carried out by the practice nurse responsible for the diabetes clinic, with considerable help from the computer operator, who carried out the clinical record search.

Results

A comparison of the results in 1985 with those of 1989, 1991 and 1995 is shown in Table CS12.1.

Table CS12.1 Number of patients with diabetes in the practice

	1985	1989	1991	1995
Total patients[1]	156	179	205	217
Recorded prevalence (%)	1.1	1.25	1.44	1.52
Number on insulin (%)	63 (40)	64 (36)	64 (33.7)	71 (32.7)
Practice-only patients (%)[2]	92 (59)	110 (61)	126 (66.3)	139 (64)

Notes: [1]All patients of the practice with diabetes
       [2]Practice patients with diabetes looked after by the practice alone

In 1989, of the 100 patients then cared for by the practice team exclusively, 93 regularly attended the diabetes clinic; for these patients the recording of data was almost 100% (Table CS12.2). The remaining patients were mainly housebound or in sheltered housing; for them, the level of recording by the doctors was not as comprehensive as for patients attending the clinic.

The results about control were self-evident: there was more systematic recording of data concerned with control.

In addition, the doctors at that time identified six areas that had contributed to the initial success of the diabetes clinic.

1 Clear objectives had been established: to identify and register all the patients with diabetes and to provide a framework for care for those patients not attending the hospital clinic.
2 In terms of identifying patients the disease register was essential, especially for planning appointments, special checks and for audit. Initially

Table CS12.2 Practice patients with diabetes looked after by the practice team alone

	1985	1989	1991	1995
Practice-only patients (%)	92 (59)	110 (61)	126 (66.3)	139 (64)
Number (%) seen in previous 12 months for diabetes	91 (99)	107 (97)	112 (88.9)	124 (89.2)
Number with recorded eye tests in previous 12 months	26 (28)	92 (84)	97 (77)	108 (77.6)
Number with recorded feet examinations/advice/chiropody provided	No records	88 (80)	97 (77)	103 (74.1)
Number with recorded BP in previous 12 months (%)	22 (23)	99 (90)	102 (81)	108 (77.6)
Number with glycosylated protein in previous 12 months (%)	Rarely done	85 (77)	97 (77)	129 (92.8)

the practice had been able to identify 156 patients, a prevalence rate of 1.1%. The patient list was held on computer and the practice nurse was responsible for its maintenance. This had worked well.

3　Seeing and recalling patients. The separate diabetic clinic allowed better liaison with the nurse, and a new protocol was devised together with a new record sheet. All patients were given a personal record booklet which gave useful educational information. The nurse was recognized as the key worker, but patients could see their own doctor when required, and had an appointment at least annually for a medical review, including an eye examination. The audit demonstrated that patients preferred to make their next appointment when attending a clinic; the computer was helpful in identifying the occasional persistent non-attender, and for search and recall for the annual eye test.

4　An audit-friendly records format which generated simple results tables.

5　A functional team. The practice nurse had been demonstrated to be invaluable: she had been able to refer directly to dietitians and chiropodists without consulting the doctors, and a constructive framework for future cooperation had been established.

6　Educating the health professionals. The continued training of the practice nurse had been beneficial. The doctors also attended diabetes symposia and subscribed to a practical journal on diabetes.

Changes resulting from the 1989 audit

The audit showed that the decision to establish a diabetes clinic had been justified. The future requirement for change would be concerned with fine tuning only.

Subsequent audits

The 1991 and 1995 audits have been helpful in several ways. For example:

1　The huge increase in the use of the glycosylated protein test as a monitoring tool is well demonstrated.

2　The apparent falling off in performance in the other variables shown in Table CS12.2 was investigated further. Two main causes were identified. The first was a failure to record clinical observations made. The second was in accuracy in the collection of the audit data. It was reassuring, therefore, that the care actually given was better than the results would suggest. Further work is being done within the practice on recording and on the rigour of audit data collection.

3 Twenty-four per cent of diabetic patients are still smoking. This subgroup is to be targeted for specific counselling.

4 Both the 1991 and the 1995 audits showed that housebound diabetic patients were most likely not to have had recent monitoring of their condition. Because this situation has not improved, practice has been changed. In future, the community nurses will monitor this group, with support from the practice nurse responsible for diabetes care.

Comment

This audit demonstrates the value of using an audit-friendly format for clinical records (*see* Chapter 7), so that data can be easily abstracted and analysed by non-medical staff. It also illustrates the value of repeated audit so that change over time, or the lack of it, can be demonstrated adequately and appropriate action taken. The principle of regular review leading to small, incremental improvement is well demonstrated.

Case Study 13

Subject of audit

PROCESS audit assessing patterns of referral practice, using practice activity analysis (*see* Chapter 7).

Background

This prospective audit was carried out in a practice with six partners in an urban area. In the same town there was a district general hospital with Accident and Emergency facilities. Moreover, the town was only 14 miles from full regional facilities, with a good road link, and from which a number of visiting consultants came for outpatient clinics, including paediatrics, dermatology and radiotherapy.

Reason for audit

A new registrar in the practice had a particular interest in referral rates. The practice was anxious that self-audit/peer view and discussion should help to reveal why referral decisions were made, and establishing an idea of current patterns would be the first step.

Aims of audit

The aim was to document the broad pattern of referrals by specialty and partner.

Method

A simple data collection sheet was devised, to be completed each time a referral letter was signed during one calender month. The limitation of measuring referral rates over a short period of time was recognized, particularly against a background of random fluctuation in patients presenting and requiring referral. The information collected included the sex and age of the patient, the hospital, specialty and consultant to whom they were referred, an indication of the urgency, and the presumptive diagnosis or presenting problem. The reason(s) for referral were indicated, with the choice from the following:

- set procedure
- known diagnosis and/or help with management
- investigation
- diagnosis
- doctor relief.

Who carried out the audit?

The registrar devised and supervised the data collection and analysis; individual partners assisted by entering the data for their own referrals on the questionnaire provided. The practice secretaries, who typed the referral letters, reminded doctors if the questionnaire was not completed.

Results

There was a total of 164 referrals over one month. The referral rates by doctor and by specialty are shown in Table CS13.1. The numbers of

Table CS13.1   Referral rates by doctor and by specialty

Specialty	Doctor							Total
	1	2	3	4	5	6	7	
Obstetrics & gynaecology	1	2	17	1	1	2	3	27
Surgery	2	3	5	2	5	2	3	21
Orthopaedics	2	0	2	6	2	1	3	16
Physiotherapy	3	0	2	3	4	1	3	16
Ophthalmology	0	3	4	1	2	2	1	13
General medicine	1	2	0	3	2	1	3	12
ENT	2	1	3	2	0	1	1	10
Dermatology	1	1	2	2	2	0	1	9
Paediatrics (inc. surgery)	0	1	2	0	1	1	3	8
Psychiatry (inc. CPNs)	2	1	2	0	2	0	1	8
Other	3	2	8	5	5	1	0	24
Total	17	16	47	25	26	12	21	164
Referral rate/100 consultations	2.5	3.7	7.4	2.9	3.3	1.6	3.6	

Average for practice   3.57

routine and urgent referrals by doctors are shown in Table CS13.2. The numbers of referrals of male and female patients are shown in Table CS13.3. The number of referrals within each referral category are shown in Table CS13.4. Doctors 1–5 were five of the six practice partners, the sixth

Table CS13.2   Numbers of routine and urgent referrals*

	Doctor							Total
	1	2	3	4	5	6	7	
Urgent	1	1	13	5	1	3	3	27
Routine	16	15	34	18	24	9	18	134
Unspecified	0	0	0	2	1	0	0	3

*Emergency referrals not included, as data collected indicated doctor with whom registered rather than referring doctor.

Table CS13.3   Number of referrals of male and female patients

Sex	Doctor							Total
	1	2	3	4	5	6	7	
Male	5	5	5	15	8	10	12	60
Female	5	11	42	10	18	2	9	97
Not specified	7	0	0	0	0	0	0	7

Table CS13.4 Number of referrals within each referral category

Reason for referral	Doctor							Total
	1	2	3	4	5	6	7	
Set procedure	4	2	11	3	7	2	1	30
Help with management	10	4	21	13	8	7	9	72
Investigation	1	2	5	6	3	0	8	25
Diagnosis	2	9	12	3	8	3	5	42
Doctor relief	1	1	2	0	0	1	0	5

being away on a sabbatical; doctor 6 was a locum and doctor 7 was the practice registrar.

One of the most striking results was the high number of gynaecological referrals, of which 63% had been referred by the one female partner (no. 3); 37.5% of the orthopaedic referrals were made by partner no. 4, who had a particular interest in rheumatology.

Given that the numbers were small, the results tended to suggest that although there was a fairly marked difference in referral rates by individual partners within the practice, putative reasons for the differences, including the types of patients consulting particular doctors with specific problems, could include the sex, age, personality and experience of the doctors concerned.

The high percentage of gynaecological referrals made by the female doctor, and of orthopaedic referrals made by doctor no. 4, reflects the special interests within the practice. Experience in a particular specialty leads to a higher rate of referral to that specialty.

Changes resulting from audit

The audit revealed some patterns and trends in referral patterns that could be pursued. It stimulated discussion on the possibility of reducing unnecessary hospital referrals by adopting referral between partners.

Was the audit repeated?

The practice is planning further work on referrals.

1 To develop a minimum data set on hospital referrals.
2 The prospective examination of a sample of records, together with doctor interviews, to discover more about the factors that influence a doctors' decision to refer.
3 To try and develop explicit criteria for referral.

Comment

The value of this exploratory audit lies in the further questions it raised among the partners about hospital referrals. It demonstrates the value of a short-term exploratory approach, gathering data sufficient to test the data collection instruments before further use.

Practice activity analysis audits involving short-term data collection and analysis are particularly suitable projects for registrars, as they can be completed within their relatively short period of attachment to a practice.

Case Study 14

Subject of audit

IMPROVING the effectiveness and efficiency of rubella immunization using a process audit.

Background

Rubella infection during pregnancy can cause severe congenital abnormality in the baby. In England and Wales in 1986 there were 196 confirmed cases of rubella infection in pregnancy.[1] Many of the pregnancies were terminated.

In any district the DHA has responsibility for rubella immunization of schoolgirls. If parents choose to have their child immunized by the general practitioner and not the DHA, the practice does not always know that it is responsible. Moreover, as the DHA does not always inform the practice when it immunizes a schoolgirl, practice records may be incomplete.

Reason for the audit

Partners were aware that some of their female patients, certain of whom had not been schoolgirls in their district, were having their first test for rubella immunity as part of routine blood testing during their first pregnancy, which is too late.

Previous practice policy was to test all women for rubella immunity when they attended for contraceptive advice and to record rubella status on the patients' manual records. The partners and practice administrator thought that policy and implementation were inadequate, but did not know to what extent. In addition the retrieval of information from manual records was sometimes difficult.

For nine months the partners had been transferring data on to a practice computer on an 'opportunistic' basis, i.e. as patients attended. From a starting point of zero records, they did not know what they had achieved.

Aims of audit

1 To determine the percentage of schoolgirls aged 13 years on the practice list who had been immunized against rubella, to compare the figure with national and local averages, and to agree upon measures that would improve uptake.
2 To determine the percentage of women aged 16–39 years who had not been sterilized, or who had had a hysterectomy, whose rubella status was recorded on the practice computer (practice policy).
3 To agree upon necessary steps to improve the testing and recording of rubella status.

Success was ascertained by comparing practice schoolgirl immunization figure with DHA and UK averages; rubella status figures were compared with the target of 100% recorded immunity for women aged 16–39 years at risk of pregnancy.

Methods

The practice administrator undertook a computer search to identify school-girls born in 1977, and identified who had had immunizations recorded. He then compared these data with the DHA records of rubella immunization of the same girls.

For the rubella status audit of women aged 16–39 years, the practice administrator undertook four computer searches, for the total number; rubella status; hysterectomy history; and sterilization history.

Who carried out the audit?

The audit was designed by the partner, who took overall responsibility, but it was carried out by the practice administrator.

Results

Immunization of schoolgirls

The results showed that immunization levels for schoolgirls were below the national and district average (Table CS14.1). The disparity between DHA figures for uptake of immunization in the practice and in the district is surprising, because the DHA is responsible for both. This difference may reflect the small number of girls being immunized in the practice, or cast doubt on the high 97% uptake for the district. As the practice team achieves its other immunization targets, there is no reason to suspect unusually poor compliance in the practice population.

Although the denominators are slightly different for the practice and the DHA and UK (girls born in 1977 for the practice; girls who have reached their 14th birthday for DHA and UK figures), analysis of the data revealed that this difference did not affect the results.

Recording of rubella status ages 16–39 years

The results of audit of rubella status reflect nine months' work recording rubella status; after a further six weeks, the rate of recording increased from 34.5% in nine months (3.8% per month) to 8.5% in six weeks (6.1% per month) (Table CS14.2).

The data do not permit distinction between lack of testing and lack of recording. As the figures for hysterectomy had already been scrutinized as part of the cervical cytology screening programme, they were more likely to be complete than figures for sterilization and rubella status.

The results answer the question posed. The practice team was able to

Table CS14.1 Immunization of girls aged 13 years (all born in 1977)

	No.	%
Total	26	
Number shown on practice computer as having been vaccinated	20	77
Number shown on DHA computer as having been vaccinated	21	81
DHA average		97*
UK average		86*

*Uptake in girls by 14th birthday.

Table CS14.2   Rubella status in women aged 16–39 years

	No.	%	No. at 6 weeks	%
Total	758		752	
Number recorded as having had hysterectomy	9		9	
Number recorded as having been sterilized	8		9	
Number of women aged 16–39 years who had no computer record of sterilization or hysterectomy	741		734	
Of this group, number whose rubella status was recorded	256	34.5	316	43

compare its results with local and national figures and identify opportunities for improvement.

Changes resulting from audit

At a practice meeting following the baseline audits of girls and women, the following changes were agreed:

1 In addition to DHA policy, the practice would attempt to ensure that every girl registered with the practice was immunized against rubella before her 14th birthday.
2 The practice administrator would regularly monitor immunization of 13-year-old girls, obtaining DHA information where necessary. It is also his responsibility to ensure that girls who have not been immunized are offered immunization, and that partners follow up defaulters.
3 All women in the age group 16–39 years should have recorded on the practice computer that they have had a hysterectomy, been sterilized or are rubella immune. It is the responsibility of the doctor or nurse who last saw the patient to ensure that the necessary recording or testing is carried out.
4 All women in the age group 16–39 years who have not had a hysterectomy or been sterilized, and whose rubella status is unknown, should be offered testing on an opportunistic basis. If they decline testing, this should be clearly noted.

Was the audit repeated?

The audit will be repeated in one year, during which period continued progress is anticipated.

Comment

The overall aim of reducing the risk of a child being born with congenital rubella syndrome is worthwhile on both humane and economic grounds.

The ultimate outcome of the success of a rubella immunization programme would be to count the number of babies affected by congenital rubella syndrome and the number of terminations performed owing to rubella infection during pregnancy. Although such an audit might be useful on a national or regional scale, it would be of little value to an individual practice in which there had been few cases per year for many years. Owing to the small denominator, measures of intermediate outcome were selected for which a standard could be set and progress measured.

The results enabled the partners and practice administrator to identify weaknesses (e.g. the transfer of information from the DHA and the follow-up of immunization defaulters) and to decide upon measures to achieve the agreed standards. The practice team could also assess the progress made in entering information into a relatively new computer system.

Although the results show that work needs to be done to implement the practice's own standards, procedures have been agreed upon and progress assessed.

Case Study 15

Subject of audit

THE audits of the care of patients with diabetes in a general practice were intended to improve glycaemic control and thereby reduce the risk of complications.

Background

Three audits were carried out in a practice of 4500 patients with 47 known patients with diabetes (1.1% of the practice population); 12 patients who regularly attend a consultant diabetic clinic were excluded.

With approximately two new cases diagnosed each year and a fairly stable population (total practice turnover of patients 5% per annum), the group of patients studied, i.e. the denominator, remained reasonably constant.

The first audit led to the partners defining a protocol for the care of patients (Appendix 1) and agreeing that they would continue to see patients with diabetes during regular surgery sessions. The second audit, a year later, led to the institution of a regular practice diabetes clinic and a new protocol (Appendix 2). The third audit reviewed the glycaemic control of patients attending the diabetes clinic.

Reasons for the audit

The first audit had shown that glycaemic control of practice patients with diabetes was unsatisfactory, and that important observations (e.g. weight, smoking history, fundoscopy and foot examination) were either not being carried out or not being recorded. The second audit showed that the first protocol did not produce much improvement.

Aim of the audit

The aim was to see how closely the practice team complied with its protocol for the care of patients with diabetes, and to assess the effectiveness of the diabetes clinic.

The audit measured the percentage of patients for whom essential data were recorded at least annually, and compared three parameters (blood pressure, glycosylated haemoglobin and weight) against ideal levels.

Methods

Patients suffering from diabetes were identified from the practice disease index. To ensure that the list was complete, a computer search was also carried out to find all patients receiving prescriptions for insulin, oral hypoglycaemic agents, Diastix (urine glucose testing sticks) and blood glucose monitoring equipment.

To ensure consistency, one partner reviewed the records of every patient with diabetes for each of the three audits. A dedicated diabetes record card had been introduced into each patient's notes when the clinic was started, so these were easy to count.

Who carried out the audit?

The partner responsible for the organization and effectiveness of the care of patients with diabetes, and now responsible for the diabetes clinic, was responsible for the audit. (Now that systems are established for recording data and less searching of records is necessary, it should be possible to delegate further audits to practice staff.)

Results

The results of data recording for the three audits are given in Table CS15.1. The relevant audit periods are year 1 (before protocol agreed), year 2 (before clinic established), and year 3 (clinic running).

Intermediate outcome measurements of clinical management between year 2 and year 3 (i.e. before and after the commencement of the diabetes clinic) are shown in Table CS15.2.

The results show that the first set of criteria and standards did not result in much improvement in the process of care, as measured by the recorded data: there were fewer recordings of examination of patients' feet for evidence of complications.

However, the third audit revealed a considerable improvement in recording once the diabetes clinic had been established, a revised protocol agreed upon and care shared with a nurse, dietitian and chiropodist. Despite this apparent improvement in process, changes in intermediate outcome measures (glycosylated haemoglobin, weight and blood pressure) were disappointing.

Table CS15.1 Data from all three audits

| | Percentage recorded | | |
	Year 1	Year 2	Year 3
1 Evidence of diagnosis	91	100	100
2 Ideal weight	12	12	100
3 Diet	21	21	100
4 Smoking history	14	14	100
5 Treatment	97	97	100
6 Visual acuity	2	20	96
7 Appearance of optic fundi	12	24	96
8 Foot examination	25	16	96
9 Urinalysis	51	60	96
10 Random blood glucose*	57	56	0
11 Glycosylated Hb	40	68	96
12 Weight	34	56	96
13 Blood pressure	76	84	96

*Random blood glucose deleted from the statement of practice policy, as glycosylated Hb gives more useful information.

Table CS15.2   Intermediate outcome measures of clinical management between year 2 and year 3

	Worse	No change	Improvement
Glycosylated Hb	57%	22%	21%
Weight	31%	19%	50%
Blood pressure	41%	39%	20%

Changes resulting from audit

Following the third and most recent audit, the doctors, nurse, dietitian and chiropodist reviewed the data and decided to take a more aggressive approach towards dietary advice, hypoglycaemic therapy and blood pressure control. The success (or otherwise) of this policy will be revealed by the next audit.

Comment

This is an example of an audit of chronic disease management using data from the clinical record (*see* Chapter 7). The same format could be used to audit other chronic conditions, such as asthma and hypertension.

In this case, outcome could have been audited by measuring the prevalence and severity of complications (which will be done), but numbers are small and the results will be subject to wide statistical error. For example, visual acuity could be compared yearly, or the number of digits possessed by each patient could be counted and compared with the number possessed last year. Frequency of hospitalization or hypoglycaemia could also be measured.

However, it is easy to record data and do nothing about them. The blood pressure of the entire practice population may be recorded, but unless those patients with abnormal levels are investigated and treated their risk of complications will not be reduced. Similarly, taking blood to test for glycosylated haemoglobin and recording the result does not reduce a diabetic patient's chance of becoming blind. These particular audits of diabetes are an example of a pleasing process audit hiding unsatisfactory intermediate outcome results (*see* Chapter 3).

Appendix CS15.1: Diabetic protocol (written after first audit)

Protocol for recording

The following data should be recorded in the note of all patients of diabetes.

Recorded once

- Evidence of diagnosis
- Ideal weight
- Diet (CHO)
- Smoking history

Recorded within the last year

- Description of treatment
- Blood sugar
- Glycosylated haemoglobin
- Visual acuity
- Peripheral pulses
- Evidence of neuropathy
- Date and severity of last hypoglycaemic attack (particularly drivers)

Recorded each visit (for whatever reason)

- Weight
- Blood pressure
- Urine analysis

Appendix CS15.2: Diabetes protocol (written after second audit)

Protocol for diabetes clinic

1 Timing
Clinic held third Tuesday every month 3.00–6.00 pm.
Annual 30-minute appointment.

2 Patients
All patients with diabetes not regularly seen at a hospital diabetic clinic.

3 Nurse
Record on green card:
- Date
- Height
- Weight
- Ideal weight (see obesity protocol for ideal weights)
- Corrected visual acuity, each eye
- Urine test for glucose, protein, blood, ketones

Arrange MSU if urine shows protein or blood
Complete green biochemistry card, ticking glycosylated haemoglobin and creatinine.

Dilate pupils
Instil 1 drop 0.5% tropicamide into each eye unless there is a dense cataract, glaucoma, history of eye surgery, pain or redness.
Consult doctor if unsure.

4 Doctor
Record on green card:

Blood pressure (see centile chart)
Condition of leg and foot pulses
Knee, ankle and plantar reflexes
Vibration and light touch senses knees, ankles and feet
Condition of fundi, particularly signs of retinopathy
Presence and severity of cataracts
Refer to eye clinic if retinopathy seen or cataract surgery necessary
Take blood for glycosylated haemoglobin and creatinine
Request random serum cholesterol if (a) not measured within past
five years or (b) previous level > 6.5 mmol/l
Reinforce general health advice (see Well Person Protocols *re* smoking, alcohol etc.)
Write to or telephone each patient when blood results are available
Note history of hypoglycaemic attacks

5 Dietitian and chiropodist
All patients should see dietitian and chiropodist each year

6 Diagnosis
Random blood glucose > 11.0 mmol/l

7 Management
Aim for random blood glucose < 10.0 mmol/l (preferably 8.0 mmol/l)
and gly Hb < 9.0%

Type I diabetes

- Refer newly diagnosed patients to consultant physician diabetes clinic for initial treatment
- Adjust insulin and diet in cooperation with dietitian
- Refer back to consultant physician diabetes clinic if control difficult or poor
- Encourage regular body mass monitoring at home

Type II diabetes (without ketonuria)

- Prescribe diet alone in first instance if weight 15% above ideal
- Repeat gly Hb and urine analysis in one month
- If uncontrolled continue dietary advice and prescribe:
  metformin 500 mg b.d. (if patient obese and serum creatinine normal); *or* gliclazide (Diamicron R 80 mg), initially 40–80 mg daily (maximum 320 mg, four tablets daily)
- Do not change an existing patient from glibenclamide (maximum 15 mg, three tablets daily) to gliclazide unless he/she has hypoglycaemic symptoms
- Consider referral to consultant physician diabetes clinic if glycosylated haemoglobin remains > 9.0%

References

Chapter 1

1 Irvine DH and Irvine S (1996) *The practice of quality*. Radcliffe Medical Press, Oxford.

Chapter 2

1 Secretaries of State for Health, Social Services, Wales, Northern Ireland and Scotland (1989) *Working for patients* (Cmd 555). HMSO, London.
2 National Health Service Executive (1996) *Promoting clinical effectiveness: a framework for action in and through the NHS*. NHSE, London.
3 Welsh Office (1996) *Towards evidence based practice: a clinical effectiveness initiative for Wales*. Welsh Office, Cardiff.
4 Evidence-Based Medicine Working Group (1992) Evidence-based medicine: a new approach to teaching the practice of medicine. *Journal of the American Medical Association*; **268**: 2420–5.
5 Sackett DL, Rosenberg WM, Muir-Gray JA, Haynes RB, Richardson WS (1996) *British Medical Journal* 312: 71–2.
6 General Medical Council (1995) *Duties of a doctor: good medical practice*. GMC, London.

Chapter 3

1 Royal College of General Practitioners (1985) *Quality in general practice* Policy Statement 2. RCGP, London.
2 Secretaries of State for Health, England, Wales, Northern Ireland and Scotland (1989) *Working for patients* (Cmd 555). HMSO, London.
3 Shaw C and Costain DW (1989) Guidelines for medical audit: seven principles. *British Medical Journal* 299: 498–9.
4 Hughes J and Humphrey C (1990) *Medical audit in general practice: a practical guide to the literature*. King Edward's Hospital Fund for London, London.
5 Royal College of General Practitioners (1994) *Quality and audit in general practice: meanings and definitions*. RCGP, London.
6 Irvine DH (1990) *Managing for quality in general practice*. King's Fund, London.
7 Donabedian A (1996) Evaluating the quality of medical care. *Millbank Memorial Fund Quarterly* 44: 166–204.
8 Buck C, Fry J and Irvine DH (1974) A framework for good primary care: the measurement and achievement of quality. *Journal of the Royal College of General Practitioners* 24, 599–604.

Chapter 4

1 Ashton J *et al.* (1976) An audit of deaths in general practice. *Update* 12: 1019–22.
2 Irvine DH *et al.* (1986) Educational development and evaluation research in the Northern region. In: Pendleton D, Schofield T, Marinker M (eds) *In pursuit of quality*. RCGP, London.
3 North of England Study of Standards and Performance in General Practice (1992). Medical audit in general practice. 1. Effects on doctors' clinical behaviour for common childhood conditions. *British Medical Journal* 304: 1480–4.
4 Grol R *et al.* (1988) Peer review in general practice: methods, standards, protocols. University Department of General Practice, Niemegen.
5 Grol R and Lawrence M (1995) *Quality improvement by peer review*. Oxford General Practice Series: 32. OUP, Oxford.
6 *Report on Public Health and Medical Subjects* (1957) No. 97. HMSO, London.
7 *Report on Public Health and Medical Subjects* (1960) No. 103. HMSO, London.
8 Campling EA, Devlin HB, Hoile RW, Lunn JN (1995) Report of the national confidential enquiry into perioperative deaths 1992–93. National Confidential Enquiry into Perioperative Deaths, London.
9 NHS Management Executive (1993) *Medical audit in primary care: a collation of evaluative projects 1991–1993*. NHSE, Leeds.

Chapter 5

1 Baker R and Presley P (1990) *The practice audit plan: a handbook of medical audit*. RCGP Severn Faculty, Bristol.
2 Russell D and Russell I (1990) Statistical issues in medical audit. In: Marinker M (ed) *Medical audit in general practice*. BMJ for MSD Foundation, London.

Chapter 6

1 North of England Study of Standards and Performance in General Practice (1990) *Setting clinical standards within small groups (Vol 1). Final Report no. 40*. Health Care Research Unit, Newcastle upon Tyne.
2 Schoenbaum SC, Gottlieb LK (1990) Algorithms based on improvement of clinical quality. *British Medical Journal* 301: 1374–6.
3 British Medical Journal (1989) *Clinical algorithms: gynaecology*. BMJ, London.
4 Field MS and Lohr KN (1992) *Guidelines for clinical practice: from development to use*. National Academy Press, Washington DC.
5 Nuffield Institute for Health (1994) *Implementing clinical practice guidelines: can guidelines be used to improve practice?* Effective Health Care no. 8. NHSE, Leeds.

6 Grimshaw S and Russell I (1993) Achieving health gain through clinical guidelines. 1. Developing scientifically valid guidelines. *Quality in Health Care* 2: 243–8.

7 Royal College of General Practitioners (1995) *The development and implementation of clinical guidelines.* Report for General Practice no. 26. RCGP, London.

8 North of England evidence based guidelines development project: summary version of evidence based guideline for the primary care management of asthma in adults (1996) *British Medical Journal* 312: 762–7.

9 North of England evidence based guidelines development project: summary version of evidence based guideline for the primary care management of stable angina (1996) *British Medical Journal* 312: 827–32.

10 Royal College of General Practitioners (1996) *Clinical guidelines for the management of acute low back pain.* RCGP, London.

11 Scottish Intercollegiate Guidelines Network (1996) *Clinical guidelines: criteria for appraisal for national use.* SIGN, Edinburgh.

12 Scottish Intercollegiate Guidelines Network (1996) *National clinical guidelines on prevention of visual impairment in diabetic patients* (no. 4); *Interface between the hospital and the community: the immediate discharge document* (no. 5); Helicobacter pylori: *eradication therapy in dyspeptic disease* (no. 6).

Chapter 7

1 Crombie D and Fleming D (1988) *Practice activity analysis.* Occasional Paper 41. RCGP, London.

2 Abrahamson JH (1987) *Survey methods in community medicine.* Churchill Livingstone, London.

3 Royal College of General Practitioners (1985) *What sort of doctor?* Report from general practice No. 23. RCGP, London.

Chapter 8

1 Pringle M, Bradley CP, Carmichael CM, Wallis H, Moore A (1995) *Significant event auditing: a study of the feasibility and potential of case-based auditing in primary medical care.* Occasional Paper No. 70, RCGP, London.

2 Royal College of General Practitioners (1990) *Who killed Susan Thompson?* Video and coursebook. MSD Foundation for RCGP, London.

3 *Report on Public Health and Medical Subjects* (1957) No. 97. HMSO, London.

4 *Report on Public Health and Medical Subjects* (1960) No. 103. HMSO, London.

5 Buck C et al. (1987) *Confidential enquiry into perioperative deaths.* Nuffield Provincial Hospital Trust, London.

6 Kessner DM et al. (1973) Assessing health quality: the case for tracers. *New England Journal of Medicine* 288: 189–94.

7 Royal College of General Practitioners (1985) *What sort of doctor?* Report from general practice No. 23. RCGP, London.
8 Royal College of General Practitioners (1990) *Fellowship by assessment.* Occasional paper 50. RCGP, London.

Chapter 9

1 Dean AD *et al.* (1990) *Epilnfo, Version 5: a word processing data base and statistics program for epidemiology on microcomputers.* Centers for Disease Control, Atlanta.

Chapter 10

1 Irvine D and Irvine S (1996) *The practice of quality.* Radcliffe Medical Press, Oxford.
2 Adelaide Medical Centre Primary Health Care Team (1991) A primary health care team manifesto. *British Journal of General Practice* 41, 31–5.
3 Gregson BA *et al.* (1991) *Interprofessional collaboration between healthcare organisations.* Occasional paper 52, Royal College of General Practitioners, London.
4 Irvine D (1990) *Managing for quality in general practice.* King Edward's Hospital Fund for London, London.
5 Donaldson L (1995) Conflict, power and negotiation. *British Medical Journal* 10: 104–7.
6 Irvine D (1997) Dysfunctional doctors: the GMC's new approach. In: Rosenthal M, Lloyd Bostock S and Mulcahey L (eds) *Perspectives and medical mishaps: pieces of the puzzle.* Open University Press, Buckingham.
7 Handy C (1994) *The empty raincoat.* Hutchinson, London.
8 Hertzberg F (1966) *Work and the nature of man.* World Publishing, New York.
9 Irvine S (1995) *The management module – diploma for advanced general practice.* Newcastle University, Newcastle.
10 Pringle M *et al.* (1991) *Making sense of managing change.* Radcliffe Medical Press, Oxford.
11 Irvine S (1992) *Balancing dreams and discipline.* Royal College of General Practitioners, London.
12 Glouberman S and Mintzberg H (1994) *Managing the care of health and the care of disease.* Paper presented to King's Fund seminar, London.

Chapter 11

1 General Medical Council (1995) *Duties of a doctor: good medical practice.* GMC, London.
2 United Kingdom Council for Nursing, Midwifery and Health Visiting (1984) *Code of professional conduct for the nurse, midwife and health visitor.* UKCC, London.

3   General Medical Council (1987) *Annual report for 1986*. GMC, London.
4   Department of Health (1990) *Medical audit in the family practitioner services*. Health Circular (FP)(90)8. HMSO, London.
5   Department of Health (1991) *Medical audit in the hospital and community services*. Health Circular (91)(2). HMSO, London.

Chapter 12

1   Primary Healthcare Clinical Audit Working Group on Clinical Outcomes Group (1994) *Clinical audit in primary health care*. Department of Health, London.

Case Study 7

1   British Hypertension Society (1993) Management guidelines in essential hypertension: report of the second working party. *British Medical Journal* 306: 983–7.

Case Study 8

1   Royal College of General Practitioners (1985) *Quality in general practice*. Policy statement 2. RCGP, London.
2   Fraser RC (1992) *Clinical method: a general practice approach*. 2nd edn. Butterworth Heinemann, Oxford.
3   Drury M (1990) (ed) *The new practice manager*. Radcliffe Medical Press, Oxford.

Case Study 9

1   Sever P, Beevers G, Bulpitt C *et al*. (1993) Management guidelines in essential hypertension: report of the second working party of the British Hypertension Society. *British Medical Journal* 306: 983–7.
2   Kannel WB. Assessment of hypertension as a predictor of cardiovascular disease in the Framingham study. In: Burley DM, Birdwood GFB, Fryer JH, Taylor SH (eds) *Hypertension: its nature and treatment*. International Symposium, Malta, 1974. Ciba, Horsham.
3   Charlton BG, Calvert N, White M *et al*. (1994) Health promotion priorities for general practice: constructing and using "indicative prevalences". *British Medical Journal* 308: 1019–22.

Case Study 14

1   Department of Health and Social Security 91986) *On the state of public health: annual report of chief medical officer of DHSS*. HMSO, London.

Index